A Text Atlas of Nail Disorders
Techniques in Investigation and Diagnosis

Third edition

Robert Baran, MD
Nail Disease Centre
Cannes, France

Rodney PR Dawber, MA, MB ChB, FRCP
Consultant Dermatologist
Churchill Hospital, Oxford, UK

Eckart Haneke, MD
Klinikk Bunaes
Sandvika/Oslo, Norway

Antonella Tosti, MD
Associate Professor of Dermatology, University of Bologna
Bologna, Italy

Ivan Bristow, MSc, BSc, DPodM, MChS
Podiatrist, University College of Northampton
Northampton, UK

With contributions from

Luc Thomas, MD, PhD
Professor of Dermatology, University of Lyon, France

Jean-Luc Drapé, MD, PhD
Professor of Radiology, Hôpital Cochin, University of Paris
Paris, France

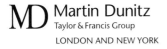
Martin Dunitz
Taylor & Francis Group
LONDON AND NEW YORK

© 1990, 1996, 2003, Martin Dunitz, a member of the Taylor & Francis Group

First published in the United Kingdom in 1990
by Martin Dunitz, Taylor & Francis Group plc, 11 New Fetter Lane, London EC4P 4EE

Tel: +44 (0) 20 7583 9855
Fax: +44 (0) 20 7842 2298
E-mail: info@dunitz.co.uk
Website: http://www.dunitz.co.uk

Third edition 2003

A CIP record for this book is available from the British Library.

ISBN 1 84184 096 3

Distributed in the USA by
Fulfilment Center
Taylor & Francis
10650 Tobben Drive
Independence, KY 41051, USA
Toll free tel: +1 800 634 7064
E-mail: taylorandfrancis@thomsonlearning.com

Distributed in Canada by
Taylor & Francis
74 Rolark Drive
Scarborough, Ontario M1R 4G2, Canada
Toll free tel: +1 877 226 2237
E-mail: tal_fran@istar.ca

Distributed in the rest of the world by
Thomson Publishing Services
Cheriton House
North Way
Andover, Hampshire SP10 5BE, UK
Tel: +44 (0) 1264 332424
E-mail: salesorder.tandf@thomsonpublishingservices.co.uk

Composition by Scribe Design, Gillingham, Kent, UK
Printed and bound in Spain by Grafos S.A. Arte Sobre Papel

Contents

List of contributors   v

Preface   vii

1 Science of the nail apparatus   1
Rodney PR Dawber

2 Nail configuration abnormalities   9
Antonella Tosti, Robert Baran, Rodney PR Dawber, Eckart Haneke

3 Modifications of the nail surface   45
Antonella Tosti, Robert Baran, Rodney PR Dawber, Eckart Haneke

4 Nail plate and soft tissue abnormalities   63
Robert Baran, Rodney PR Dawber, Eckart Haneke, Antonella Tosti

5 Periungual tissue disorders   81
Robert Baran

6 Nail consistency   121
Robert Baran, Rodney PR Dawber, Eckart Haneke, Antonella Tosti

7 Nail colour changes (chromonychia)   127
Eckart Haneke, Robert Baran, Rodney PR Dawber, Antonella Tosti

8 Onychomycosis and its treatment   143
Antonella Tosti, Robert Baran, Rodney PR Dawber, Eckart Haneke

9 Traumatic disorders of the nail   159
Rodney PR Dawber and Ivan Bristow

10 Histopathology of common nail conditions   191
Eckart Haneke

11 Ultrasonography and magnetic resonance imaging of the perionychium   201
Jean-Luc Drapé, Sophie Goettmann, Alain Chevrot and Jacques Bittoun

12 Dermatoscopy of nail pigmentation   217
Luc Thomas and Sandra Ronger

13 Treatment of common nail disorders   225
Antonella Tosti, Robert Baran, Rodney PR Dawber, Eckart Haneke

Index   235

List of contributors

Robert Baran, MD
Nail Disease Centre
42 rue des Serbes
06400 Cannes, France

Jacques Bittoun, MD, PhD
Centre Inter Etablissements de Résonance
Magnétique (CIERM)
CHU de Bicêtre
Université Paris Sud
74 rue du general Leclerc
94274 Le Kremlin-Bicêtre Cedex, France

Ivan Bristow, MSc, BSc, DPodM, MChS
School of Podiatry
University College of Northampton
Park Campus
Northampton NN2 7AL, UK

Alain Chevrot, MD
Service de Radiologie B
Hôpital Cochin
27 rue du Faubourg Saint-Jacques
75679 Paris Cedex 14, France

Rodney PR Dawber, MA, MB ChB, FRCP
Department of Dermatology
Churchill Hospital
Old Road
Oxford OX3 7LJ, UK

Jean-Luc Drapé, MD, PhD
Service de Radiologie B
Hôpital Cochin
27 rue du faubourg Saint-Jacques
75679 Paris Cedex 14, France

Sophie Goettmann, MD
Service de Dermatologie
Hôpital Bichat
46 rue Henri Huchard
75018 Paris, France

Eckart Haneke, MD
Klinikk Bunaes
Løkkeåsveien 3
1300 Sandvika / Oslo, Norway

Sandra Ronger, MD, PhD
Unité Dermatologique
Hôtel Dieux
69288 Lyon Cedex 02, France

Luc Thomas, MD, PhD
Unité Dermatologique
Hôtel Dieux
69288 Lyon Cedex 02, France

Antonella Tosti, MD
Istituto di Clinica Dermatologica
Università di Bologna
Policlinico S Orsola
Via G Massarenti 1
40138 Bologna, Italy

Preface

The editorial team were reassured that the second edition, with its differential diagnostic style of presenting clinical information together with liberal use of colour illustrations, had been successful enough to merit a further edition. Seven years have passed since the previous edition and evidently, like for other areas of clinical medicine, diagnostic and therapeutic advances have been made in relation to nail disorders. These are reflected in this third edition.

The science of the nail apparatus and the clinical management of the foot and traumatic nail disorders are now much more closely allied to podiatry and this is shown in the contributions of Ivan Bristow and by his inclusion as a member of the editorial team.

Until relatively recently only mycological and histological diagnostic routines were used to investigate nail diseases. Luc Thomas and Sandra Ronger have contributed a new section on the use of dermatoscopy in the nail and periungual tissues, reflecting the increasing subtlety of this technique in the diagnosis of pigmentary conditions.

Ultrasonography and Magnetic Resonance Imaging (MRI) have become very important in diagnosis and presurgical assessment and a contribution by Jean-Luc Drape shows the advances in this field.

Many of our dermatological and podiatric colleagues use this book as their main diagnostic tool and to further aid our readers we have increased the number of 'further reading' references throughout the book.

Robert Baran
Rodney PR Dawber
Eckart Haneke
Antonella Tosti
Ivan Bristow

January 2003

1 Science of the nail apparatus

Rodney PR Dawber

Structure • Microscopic anatomy • Blood and nerve supply • Nail dynamics • The nails in childhood and old age

The anatomy and physiology of the nail apparatus on the hand may be considered in isolation; however, the nail apparatus on the toes must always be considered in relation to toe and foot structure and function. Many disorders of nails are directly due to functional faults in the foot; alternatively, diseases of the nail apparatus may be modified by alterations in digital or foot shape or movement (see Chapter 9).

> **The nail is an important 'tool' and adds subtlety and protection to the digit**

The nail apparatus develops from the primitive epidermis. Its main function is to produce a strong, relatively inflexible nail plate over the dorsal surface of the end of each digit. The nail plate acts as a protective covering for the digit by exerting counter-pressure over the volar skin and pulp; its relative flatness adds to the precision and delicacy of the ability to pick up small objects and of many other subtle finger functions. Counter-pressure against the plantar skin and pulp prevents the 'heaping up' of the distal soft tissue. Finger nails typically cover approximately one-fifth of the dorsal surface, while on the great toe, the nail may cover up to half of the dorsum of the digit. Toe nails and finger nails have varying shapes and curvature. This is controlled by many factors: the area of the proximal matrix; the rate of cell division within it; and the shape of the underlying distal phalanx to which the nail is firmly attached by vertical connective tissue.

STRUCTURE

The component parts of the nail apparatus are shown in Figure 1.1. The rectangular nail plate is the largest structure, resting on and firmly attached to the nail bed and the underlying bones; it is less firmly attached proximally, apart from the posterolateral corners. Approximately one-quarter of the nail is covered by the proximal nail fold, while a narrow margin of the sides of the nail plate is often occluded by the lateral nail folds. Underlying the proximal part of the nail is the white lunula ('half-moon' or lunule); this area represents the most distal region of the matrix. The natural shape of the free margin of the nail is the same as the contour of the distal border of the lunula. The nail plate distal to the lunula is usually pink owing to its translucency, which allows the redness of the vascular nail bed to be seen through it. The proximal nail fold has

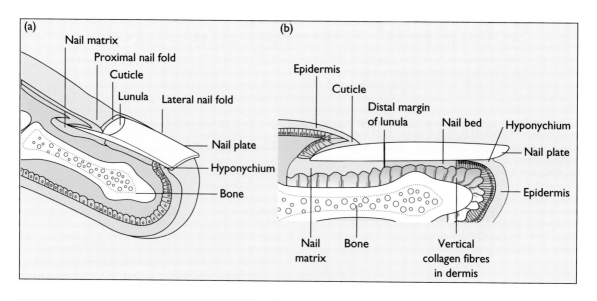

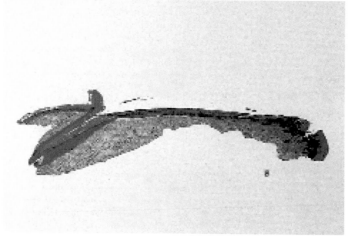

Figure 1.1
(a), (b) Nail apparatus structures;
(c) longitudinal nail biopsy section,
oriented to equate with (b).

(c)

two epithelial surfaces, dorsal and ventral; at the junction of the two the cuticle projects distally on to the nail surface. The lateral nail folds are in continuity with the skin on the sides of the digit laterally, and medially they are joined by the nail bed.

The nail matrix can be subdivided into proximal (or dorsal) and distal (or intermediate) sections, the latter underlying the nail plate to the distal border of the lunula. It is now generally considered that the nail bed contributes to the deep surface of the nail plate (ventral matrix), although this thin, soft, deep component plays little part in the functional integrity of the nail plate in its distal part. At the point of separation of the nail plate from the nail bed, the proximal part of the hyponychium may be modified as the solehorn. In hooved animals this is the site of hard keratin hoof formation – it may also be the source of hard, distal subungual hyperkeratosis in diseases such as psoriasis and pachyonychia congenita. Beyond the solehorn region the hyponychium terminates at the distal nail groove; the tip of the digit beyond this ridge assumes the structure of the epidermis elsewhere.

When the attached nail plate is viewed from above, several distinct areas may be visible, such as the proximal lunula and the larger pink zone. On close examination two further distal zones can often be identified: the distal yellowish-white margin, and immediately proximal to this the onychodermal band. The latter is a barely perceptible, narrow transverse band 0.5–1.5 mm wide. The exact anatomical basis for the onychodermal (onychocorneal) band is not known but it appears to have a separate blood supply from that of the main body of the nail bed; if the tip of the finger is pressed firmly, the band and an area just proximal to it blanch, and if the pressure is repeated several times the band reddens.

MICROSCOPIC ANATOMY

Nail fold

The proximal nail fold is similar in structure to the adjacent skin but is normally devoid of dermatoglyphic markings and sebaceous glands. From the distal area of the proximal nail fold the cuticle reflects on to the surface of the nail plate. The cuticle is composed of modified stratum corneum and serves to protect the structures at the base of the nail, particularly the germinative matrix, from environmental insults such as irritants, allergens and bacterial and fungal pathogens.

Nail matrix

The proximal (dorsal) and distal (intermediate) nail matrix produces the major part of the nail plate. Like the epidermis of the skin, the matrix possesses a dividing basal layer producing keratinocytes; these differentiate, harden, die and contribute to the nail plate, which is thus analogous to the epidermal stratum corneum. The nail matrix keratinocytes mature and keratinize without keratohyalin (granular layer) formation. Apart from this, the detailed cytological changes seen in the matrix epithelium under the electron microscope are essentially the same as in the epidermis.

The nail matrix contains melanocytes in the lowest two cell layers and these donate pigment to keratinocytes. Under normal circumstances pigment is not visible in the nail plate of white individuals, but many black people show patchy melanogenesis as linear longitudinal pigmented bands.

> **On the great toes, the nail matrix sits like a saddle on the distal phalanx**

Nail bed

The nail bed consists of an epidermal part and an underlying dermal part closely apposed to the periosteum of the distal phalanx. There is no subcutaneous fat layer in the nail bed, although scattered dermal fat cells may be visible microscopically. The epidermal layer is usually no more than two or three cells thick, and the transitional zone from living keratinocyte to dead ventral nail plate cell is abrupt, occurring in the space of one horizontal cell layer. As the cells differentiate they are incorporated into the ventral surface of the nail plate and move distally with this layer.

The nail bed dermal fibrous tissue network is mainly oriented vertically, being directly attached to phalangeal periosteum and the epidermal basal lamina. Within the connective tissue network lie blood vessels, lymphatics, a fine network of elastic fibres and scattered fat cells; at the distal margin, eccrine sweat glands have been seen.

Nail plate

The nail plate is composed of three horizontal layers: a thin dorsal lamina, the thicker intermediate lamina and a ventral layer from the nail bed. Microscopically it consists of flattened, dead squamous cells closely apposed to each other. In older people acidophilic masses are occasionally seen, called 'pertinax bodies'.

The nail plate is rich in calcium, found as the phosphate in hydroxyapatite crystals; it is bound to phospholipids intracellularly. The relevance of other elements which are present in smaller amounts, such as copper, manganese, zinc and iron, is not exactly known. Calcium exists in a concentration of 0.1% by weight, 10 times greater than in hair. Calcium does not significantly contribute to the hardness of the nail. Nail hardness is mainly due to dense sulphur protein from the matrix, which contrasts with the relatively soft keratin of the epidermis. The normal curvature of the nail relates to the shape of the underlying phalangeal bone to which the nail plate is directly bonded via the vertical connective tissue attachment between the subungual epithelium and the periosteum.

BLOOD AND NERVE SUPPLY

> **The nail apparatus has a magnificent blood supply with many anastomoses**

There is a rich arterial blood supply to the nail bed and matrix derived from paired digital arteries (Figure 1.2). The main supply passes into the pulp space of the distal phalanx before reaching the dorsum of the digit. The volar digital nerves (Figure 1.2c) are similarly important in providing nerves to the deep nail apparatus structures. An accessory blood supply arises further back on the digit and does not enter the pulp space. There are two main arterial arches (proximal and distal) supplying the nail bed and matrix, formed from anastomoses of the branches of the digital arteries. In the event of damage to the main supply in the pulp space, such as might occur with trauma, infection or scleroderma, there may be sufficient blood from the accessory vessels to permit normal growth of the nail.

There is a capillary loop system to the whole of the nail fold, but the loops to the roof and matrix are flatter than those below the exposed nail. There are many arteriovenous anastomoses below the nail – glomus bodies, which are concerned with heat regulation. Glomus bodies are important in maintaining acral circulation under cold conditions – arterioles constrict with cold, but glomus bodies dilate. The nail beds of fingers and toes contain such bodies (93–501 per cm^2). Each glomus is an encapsulated oval organ 300 μm long, made up of a tortuous vessel uniting an artery and venule, a nerve supply and a capsule; also within the capsules are many cholinergic muscle cells.

NAIL DYNAMICS

Clinicians used to observing the slow rate of clearance of diseased or damaged nails are apt to view the nail apparatus as a rather inert structure, although it is in fact the centre of marked kinetic and biochemical activity.

Cell kinetics

Unlike the hair matrix, which undergoes a resting or quiescent (telogen) phase every few years, the nail matrix germinative layers

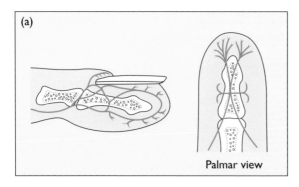

Palmar view

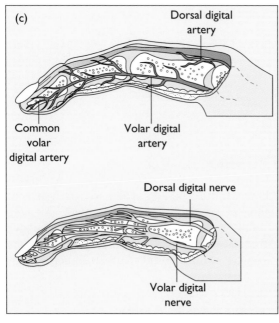

Dorsal digital artery

Common volar digital artery

Volar digital artery

Dorsal digital nerve

Volar digital nerve

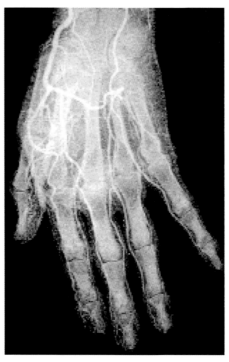

(b)

Figure 1.2
Digital blood and nerve supply: (a) showing arterial anastomoses; (b) arterial supply from hand to digits (radio-opaque dye seen in arteries); (c) major digital arteries and nerve supply.

continue to undertake DNA synthesis, to divide and to differentiate throughout life, akin to the epidermis in this respect. Exactly which parts of the nail apparatus contribute to the nail plate has been debated; it is now usually accepted that the three-layer nail plate is produced from the proximal matrix, the distal matrix and the nail bed (sterile ventral matrix).

The nail grows continuously through-out life

Why the nail grows flat, rather than as a heaped-up keratinous mass, has generated much thought and discussion. Several factors probably combine to produce a relatively flat nail plate; the orientation of the matrix rete pegs and papillae, the direction of cell differentiation, and the fact that since keratinization takes place within the confines of the nail base, limited by the proximal nail fold dorsally and the terminal phalanx ventrally, the differentiating cells can only move distally and form a flat structure – by the time they leave the confines of the proximal nail fold all the cells are dead, keratinized and hardened.

Linear nail growth

Many studies have investigated the linear growth rates of the nail plate in health and disease; their findings are summarized in Tables 1.1 and 1.2. Finger nails grow approximately 1 cm every 3 months and toe nails at half this rate.

Table 1.1 Physiological and environmental factors affecting the rate of linear nail growth

Faster growth	Slower growth
Day-time	Night-time
Pregnancy	First day of life
Minor trauma/nail biting	
Right-hand nails	Left-hand nails
Youth, increasing age	Old age
Fingers	Toes
Summer	Winter or cold environment
Middle, ring and index fingers	Thumb and little finger
Male (?)	Female (?)

THE NAILS IN CHILDHOOD AND OLD AGE

Childhood

In early childhood, the nail plate is thin and may show temporary koilonychia. Because of the shape of the matrix, some children show ridges that start laterally by the proximal nail fold and join at a central point just short of the free margin, to give a 'herringbone' arrangement of the ridges (chevron nails). In one study 92% of normal infants aged 8–9 weeks showed a single transverse line (Beau's line) on the finger nails. One child demonstrated a transverse depression through the whole nail thickness on all 20 digits.

Old age

Many of the changes seen in old age may occur in younger age groups with impaired arterial blood supply. Elastic tissue changes diffusely affecting the nail bed epidermis are often seen histologically; these changes may

Table 1.2 Pathological factors affecting the rate of linear nail growth

Faster growth	Slower growth
Psoriasis	Finger immobilization
normal nails	Fever
pitting	Beau's lines
onycholysis	Denervation
Pityriasis rubra pilaris	Poor nutrition
Idiopathic onycholysis of women	Kwashiorkor
Bullous ichthyosiform erythroderma	Hypothyroidism
Hyperthyroidism	Yellow nail syndrome
Drugs	Relapsing polychondritis
Arteriovenous shunts	

be due to the effects of ultraviolet (UV) radiation, although it has been stated that the nail plate is an efficient filter of UVB radiation. The whole subungual area in old age may show thickening of blood vessel walls with vascular elastic tissue fragmentation. Pertinax bodies are often seen in the nail plate; they are probably remnants of nuclei of keratinocytes. Nail growth is inversely proportional to age; related to this slower growth, corneocytes are larger in old age. Since nails tend to thicken with age and some diseases, it may well be that the volume of nail production per unit of time does not change.

The nail plate becomes paler, dull and opaque with advancing years and white nails similar to those seen in cirrhosis, uraemia and hypoalbuminaemia may be seen in normal individuals. Longitudinal ridging is present to some degree in most people after 50 years of age and this may give a 'sausage links' appearance.

2 Nail configuration abnormalities

Antonella Tosti, Robert Baran, Rodney PR Dawber, Eckart Haneke

Clubbing (Hippocratic fingers) • Koilonychia • Transverse overcurvature • Dolichonychia (long nails) • Brachyonychia (short nails) • Parrot-beak nails • Round fingerpad • Hook and claw-like nails • Micronychia, macronychia and polydactyly • Worn-down, shiny nails • Anonychia and onychatrophy • Further reading

CLUBBING (HIPPOCRATIC FINGERS)

The bulbous digital deformity known as clubbing (Figure 2.1a,b) was described as early as the fifth century BC when Hippocrates noted such changes in patients suffering from empyema. The diagnostic signs comprise:

1 Overcurvature of the nails in the proximal to distal and transverse planes (Figure 2.2).
2 Enlargement of periungual soft tissue structures confined to the tip of each digit.

A simple method to detect clubbing is measurement of the phalangeal depth ratio (Figure 2.3). In a normal finger the distal phalangeal depth is smaller than the interphalangeal depth. In clubbing this relationship is reversed (> 1). The measurement can easily be taken using a caliper in less than a minute.

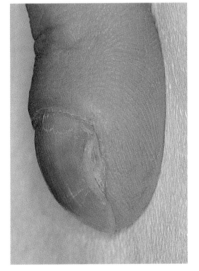

(a)

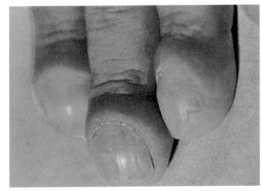

(b)

Figure 2.1
(a, b) Clubbing.

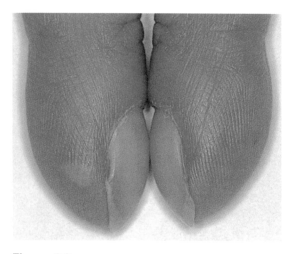

Figure 2.2
Clubbing, demonstrating typical nail curvature and obliteration of the 'window'.

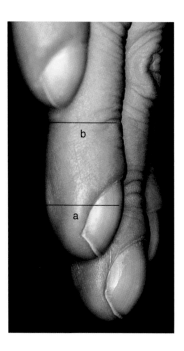

Figure 2.3
In clubbing the phalangeal depth ratio is greater than 1. (a/b >1)

The increased nail curvature usually affects all 20 digits, but may be particularly obvious on the thumbs, index and middle fingers. The 'watch-glass' shape of the nail may occur as

an isolated deformity without any associated enlargement of the tip of the digit. The shape of the curved nails is variable and may appear fusiform, like a bird's beak, or clubbed like a watch-glass. The matrix quite often appears abnormally large. There are three main types of clubbing:

1 Simple clubbing.
2 Hypertrophic pulmonary osteoarthropathy.
3 Pachydermoperiostosis.

Simple clubbing

Simple clubbing is the most common category and has several distinctive characteristics:

1 Increased nail curvature occurs with a transverse furrow separating it from the rest of the nail both in the early stage and after resolution. The onset is usually gradual and painless, except in some cases of carcinoma of the lung in which clubbing may develop abruptly and be associated with severe pain.
2 Hypertrophy of the soft parts of the terminal segment caused by firm, elastic, oedematous infiltration of the pulp, which may spread to the dorsal surface with marked periungual swelling.
3 Hyperplasia of the dermal fibrovascular tissue may extend to involve the adjacent matrix. This accounts for one of the earliest signs of clubbing – abnormal mobility of the nail base, which can be rocked back and forth giving the impression that it is floating on a soft oedematous pad. The increased vascularity is responsible for the slow return of colour when the nail is pressed and released.
4 Acral cyanosis is often observed.

In the early stages clubbing may involve one hand only, though eventually both hands become affected symmetrically. Several stages of clubbing or acropachy may be distinguished: suspected, slight, average and severe. In practice the degree of the deformity may be gauged by Lovibond's 'profile sign' which measures the angle between the curved nail plate and the proximal nail fold when the finger is viewed from the radial aspect. This is normally 160°, but exceeds 180° in clubbing. A modified profile sign is assessed by measuring the angle between the middle and the terminal phalanx at the interphalangeal joint: in normal fingers the distal phalanx forms an almost straight (180°) extension of the middle phalanx, whereas in severe clubbing this angle may be reduced to 160° or even 140°. However, the best indicator may be the simple clinical method adopted by Schamroth: in normal individuals a distinct aperture or 'window', usually diamond-shaped, is formed at the base of the nail bed; early clubbing obliterates this window. (Fig 2.2).

Radiological changes occur in less than one-fifth of cases. These include phalangeal demineralization and irregular thickening of the cortical diaphysis. Ungual tufts generally show considerable variations and may be prominent in advanced stages of the disease. Bony atrophy may be present.

Congenital finger clubbing may be accompanied by changes such as hyperkeratosis of the palms and soles, and cortical hypertrophy of the long bones. Familial clubbing may be associated with hypertrophic osteoarthropathy; some authors regard simple clubbing as a mild form of the latter. Isolated watch-glass nails without other deformities are also constitutionally determined. Rare cases of unilateral Hippocratic nails have been reported due to obstructed circulation, oedema of the soft tissues and dystrophy of the affected parts. The pathological process apparently responsible for clubbing and its associated changes is the increased blood flow due to the opening of many anastomotic shunts.

> **Acquired clubbing almost always has an internal cause**

Hypertrophic pulmonary osteoarthropathy

This disorder is characterized by the following five signs:

1 Clubbing of the nails.
2 Hypertrophy of the upper and lower extremities similar to the deformity found in acromegaly.
3 Joint changes with pseudo-inflammatory, symmetrical, painful arthropathy of the large limb joints, especially those of the legs. This syndrome is almost pathognomonic of malignant chest tumours, especially lung carcinoma and mesothelioma of the pleura; less commonly bronchiectasis is seen. Gynaecomastia may also be present.
4 There may be bone changes such as bilateral, proliferative periostitis and moderate, diffuse decalcification.
5 Peripheral neurovascular disorders such as local cyanosis and paraesthesia are not uncommon.

Hypertrophic osteoarthropathy confined to the lower extremities appears as a manifestation of arterial graft sepsis.

Pachydermoperiostosis

Pachydermoperiostosis (idiopathic hypertrophic osteoarthropathy) is rare. In most of the reported cases the digital changes typically begin at or about the time of puberty. The

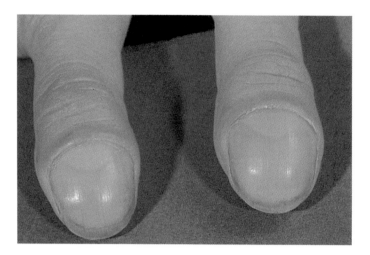

Figure 2.4
Clubbing in pachydermoperiostosis.

ends of the fingers and toes are bulbous and often grotesquely shaped, with hyperhidrosis of the hands and the feet (Figure 2.4). The clubbing stops abruptly at the distal interphalangeal joint. In this type the lesions of the finger tips are clinically identical to those of hypertrophic pulmonary osteoarthropathy. However, in pachydermoperiostosis the thickened cortex appears homogeneous on X-ray examination and does not impinge on the medullary space. Acro-osteolysis of the distal phalanges has been reported.

The pachydermal change of the extremities and face, with furrowing and oiliness of the skin, is the most characteristic feature of the disorder; it is termed the Touraine–Solente–Golé syndrome. Nevertheless, in hypertrophic pulmonary osteoarthropathy there may be facial skin and scalp changes indistinguishable from those seen in pachydermoperiostosis; this may be due to a common genetic factor. In the differential diagnosis acromegaly must be considered; this enhances tufting of the terminal phalanges and presents an anchor-like appearance, but without acro-osteolysis. Thyroid acropachy is usually associated with exophthalmos, pretibial myxoedema and abnormal thyroid function.

It should be noted that only rarely will any type of clubbing present to a dermatologist, since in most cases it is simply one sign among many relating to the primary cause.

Classification of clubbing

The principal general causes of clubbing are listed in Table 2.1; a more comprehensive list of causes is given below.

Idiopathic forms

Hereditary and congenital forms, sometimes associated with other anomalies:

- familial and genotypic pachydermoperiostosis
- racial forms (Africans)
- syndrome of pernio, periostosis and lipodystrophy
- Muckle–Wells syndrome.

Table 2.1 General causes of clubbing and pseudoclubbing

Clubbing	Pseudoclubbing

Unilateral
  Aortic/subclavian aneurysm
  Brachial plexus injury
  Trauma (Figure 2.5)
	Yellow nail syndrome (Figure 2.7)
	Gout
	Sarcoidosis
	Osteoid osteoma
	Perineurioma
	Metastases

Lower extremities Arterial graft sepsis	Congenital abnormalities Chronic paronychia – severe hook nail

General
  Congenital
    familial/sporadic
  Thoracic tumours (bronchopulmonary cancers)
  Pulmonary
  Cardiovascular
  Gastrointestinal
    inflammatory bowel disease
    parasitosis
    liver disease
    tropical sprue
  Endocrine/metabolic
    thyroid, acromegaly (Figure 2.6)
    malnutrition
  AIDS
    Secondary to pulmonary and other infections	

Acquired forms

1 Thoracic disorders are involved in about 80% of cases of clubbing, often with the common denominator of hypoxia:
   - bronchopulmonary diseases, especially chronic and infective bronchiectasis, abscess and cyst of the lung, pulmonary tuberculosis
   - sarcoidosis, pulmonary fibrosis, emphysema, Ayerza's syndrome, chronic pulmonary venous engorgement, asthma in infancy, mucoviscidosis
   - blastomycosis, pneumonia, *Pneumocystis carinii* infection, AIDS.

2 Thoracic tumours:
   - primary or metastatic bronchopulmonary cancers, pleural tumours, mediastinal tumours
   - Hodgkin's disease, lymphoma, pseudotumour due to oesophageal dilatation.

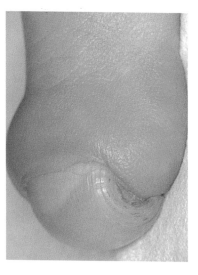

Figure 2.5
Pseudoclub-bing due to trauma – hooked nail deformity.

3 Cardiovascular disease:
- congenital heart disease associated with cyanosis (rarely non-cyanotic)
- thoracic vascular malformations; stenoses and arteriovenous aneurysms
- Osler's disease (subacute bacterial endocarditis)
- congestive cardiac failure
- myxoma
- Raynaud's disease, erythromelalgia, Maffucci's syndrome.

4 Disorders of the alimentary tract (5% of cases):
- oesophageal, gastric and colonic cancer
- disease of the small intestine

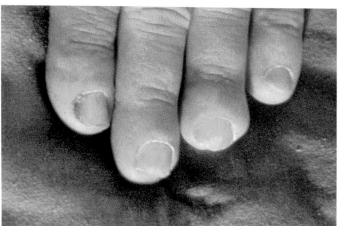

Figure 2.6
Clubbed appearance in acromegaly. (Courtesy of D. Wendling.)

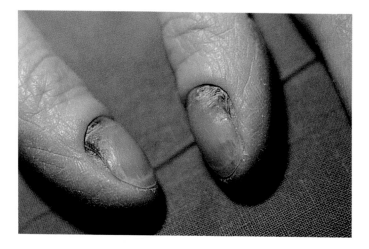

Figure 2.7
Pseudoclubbing in yellow nail syndrome.

- colonic disease
- amoebiasis and inflammatory states of the colon
- ulcerative colitis
- familial polyposis, Gardner's syndrome
- ascariasis
- active chronic hepatitis
- primary or secondary cirrhoses
- purgative abuse.

5 Endocrine origin:
- Diamond's syndrome (pretibial myxoedema, exophthalmos and finger clubbing)
- acromegaly.

6 Haematological causes:
- methaemoglobinaemia
- sulphaemoglobinaemia
- haemoglobinopathies
- primary or secondary polycythaemia associated with hypoxia
- poisoning by phosphorus, arsenic, alcohol, mercury or beryllium.

7 Hypervitaminosis A.

8 Malnutrition, kwashiorkor.

9 Addiction (hashish, heroin).

10 Syringomyelia, POEMs syndrome (peripheral neuropathy, organomegaly, endocrinopathy, monoclonal plasmaproliferative disease, skin changes).

11 Lupus erythematosus.

12 Unilateral or limited to a few digits:
- subluxation of the shoulder (with paralysis of the brachial plexus), medial nerve neuritis
- Pancoast–Tobias syndrome
- aneurysm of the aorta or the subclavian artery
- sarcoidosis
- tophaceous gout.

13 Lower extremities:
- arterial graft sepsis.

14 Isolated forms:
- local injury, whitlow, lymphangitis
- subungual epidermoid inclusions.

15 Transitory form: physiological in the newborn child (due to reversal of the circulation at birth).

16 Occupational acro-osteolysis (exposure to vinyl chloride).

KOILONYCHIA

Koilonychia (spoon-shaped nails) is the opposite of clubbing. The nail is firmly attached to bone by vertical dermal connective tissue bundles in the subungual area which bond directly to the bony periosteum. In the early stages of koilonychia there is flattening of the nail plate. Later, the edges become everted upwards and the nail appears concave, giving rise to the characteristic 'spoon' shape (Figures 2.8–2.11). In mild cases the water test may enable a drop of water to be retained on the nail plate. The subungual tissues may be normal, or affected by hyperkeratosis at the lateral and/or the distal margin.

> **Koilonychia is more often due to local rather than systemic factors**

1 In neonates and in infancy, koilonychia is a temporary physiological condition (Figures 2.12, 2.13). There is a proven correlation between koilonychia and iron deficiency (with normal haemoglobin values) in infants.

2 Koilonychia is a common manifestation of the rare Plummer–Vinson syndrome in association with anaemia, dysphagia and glossitis.

3 When subungual keratosis accompanies koilonychia, psoriasis should be considered, as well as occupational causes, which may be relevant in those who work with cement, or in car mechanics whose hands suffer constant immersion in oil, for example.

4 Koilonychia may result from thin nails of any cause (old age, peripheral arterial disease and so on).

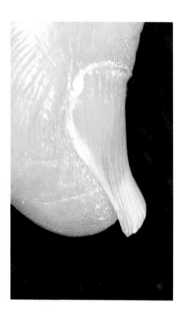

Figure 2.8
Koilonychia or 'spoon-shaped' nail; thin nail variety.

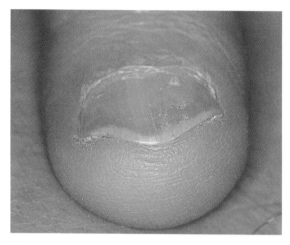

Figure 2.9
Koilonychia – distal view with some terminal traumatic whitening.

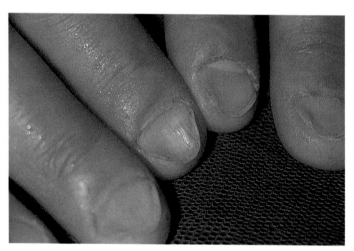

Figure 2.10
Koilonychia – severe variety, of many nails. Involvement of the first three nails is a plea for an occupational cause.

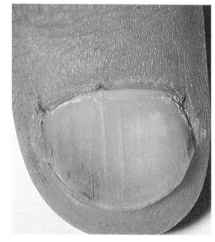

Figure 2.11
Koilonychia – transverse and longitudinal curvature evident.

5 Soft nails of any cause (mainly occupational) may also cause this condition.

6 Hereditary and congenital forms (Figures 2.14–2.16) are sometimes associated with other nail signs such as leukonychia.

The most common causes of koilonychia are probably occupational softening and iron deficiency (Table 2.2) Occupational koilonychia is often associated with mild nail-plate surface abnormalities and nail plate discoloration.

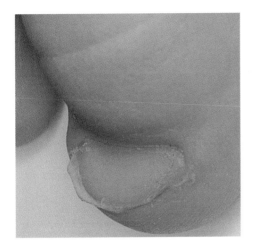

Figure 2.12
Koilonychia – temporary type of early infancy.

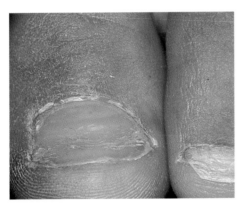

Figure 2.13
Physiological koilonychia and thinning in the toe nails of a 3-month-old infant.

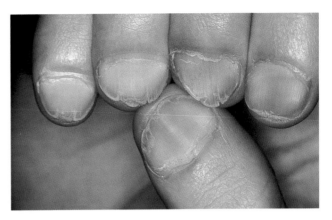

Figure 2.14
Severe congenital koilonychia.

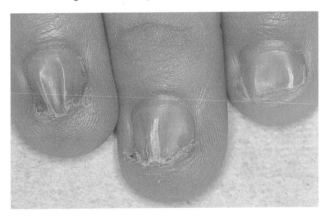

Figure 2.15
Koilonychia in hereditary ectodermal dysplasia.

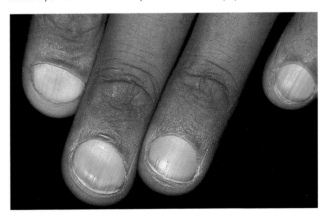

Figure 2.16
Congenital koilonychia associated with total leukonychia.

Table 2.2 Common causes of koilonychia

Physiological
> Early childhood (Figures 2.12–2.13)

Idiopathic

Congenital
> LEOPARD syndrome
> Ectodermal dysplasias (Figure 2.15)
> Trichothiodystrophy
> Nail–patella syndrome

Acquired
> Metabolic/endocrine
> > iron deficiency
> > acromegaly
> > haemochromatosis
> > porphyria
> > renal dialysis/transplant
> > thyroid disease
> Dermatoses
> > alopecia areata
> > Darier's disease
> > lichen planus
> > psoriasis
> > Raynaud's disease
> Occupational
> > contact with oils, e.g. engineering industry
> Infections
> > onychomycosis
> > syphilis
> Traumatic
> > toes of rickshaw pullers
> Carpal tunnel syndrome

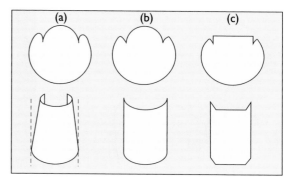

Figure 2.17
Transverse overcurvature showing the three subtypes: (a) pincer or trumpet nail; (b) tile-shaped nail; and (c) plicatured nail with sharply angled lateral margins.

Table 2.3 Common causes of transverse overcurvature

Congenital
> Hidrotic ectodermal dysplasia
> Hypohidrotic ectodermal dysplasia
> Congenital onychodysplasia of index finger nails
> Yellow nail syndrome (Figure 2.22)
> > pseudo yellow nail syndrome (insecticides and weed killers) (Figure 2.21)

Developmental
> Pincer nails (Figures 2.18, 2.19)

Acquired
> Osteoarthritis (Figure 2.18b, d)
> Neglect, e.g. of toe nails in old age

TRANSVERSE OVERCURVATURE

There are three main types of transverse overcurvature: the arched, pincer or trumpet nail; the tile-shaped nail; and a third less common variety, the 'plicatured' nail (Figure 2.17). Table 2.3 lists some of the causes of transverse overcurvature, as seen in Figures 2.18–2.23.

> **Transverse overcurvature may cause ingrowing nail of the hand**

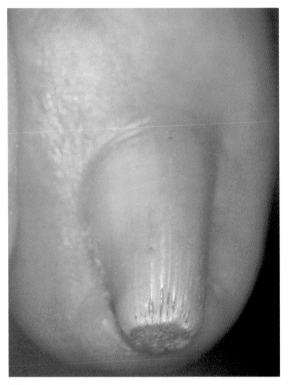

(a)

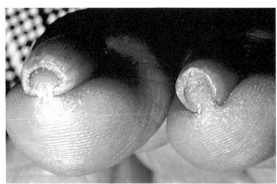

(b)

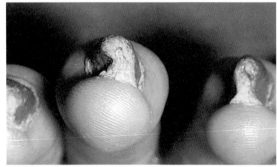

(c)

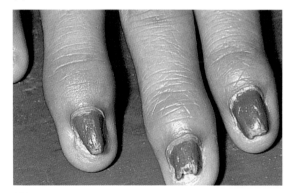

(d)

Figure 2.18
(a–d) Varying degrees of pincer nail deformity.

Pincer nail

Pincer nail is characterized by transverse overcurvature that increases along the longitudinal axis of the nail and reaches its greatest proportion towards the tip (Figures 2.18, 2.19). At this point the lateral borders tighten around the soft tissues, which are pinched without necessarily disrupting the epidermis. Eventually the soft tissue may actually disappear, sometimes accompanied by resorption of the underlying bone. Subungual exostosis may present in this way: the dorsal extension of bone producing the pincer nail (the exostosis) must be excised. The lateral borders of the nail exert a constant pressure, permanently constricting the deformed nail plate (unguis constringens). In extreme cases they may join together, forming a tunnel, or they may become rolled, taking the form of a cone. In certain varieties, the nails are shaped like claws, resembling pachyonychia congenita.

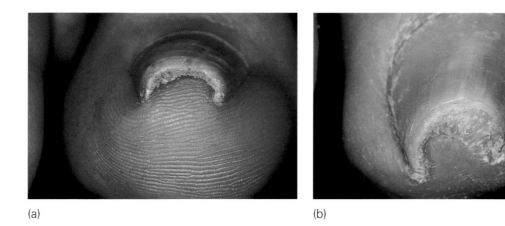

(a)   (b)

Figure 2.19
(a, b) Progressive worsening of the pincer nail deformity in 5 years.

This morphological abnormality would be no more than a curiosity if the constriction were not occasionally accompanied by pain which can be provoked by the lightest of touch, such as the weight of a bedsheet. There are a number of subtypes of this condition:

1   The inherited form usually shows symmetrical involvement of both the great toe nails and of the lesser toe nails. The great toe nails typically have lateral deviation of their longitudinal axis, the lesser toe nails being deviated medially. This dystrophy is a

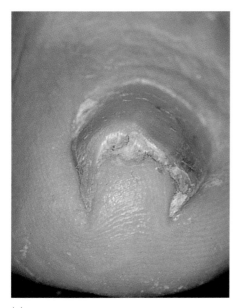

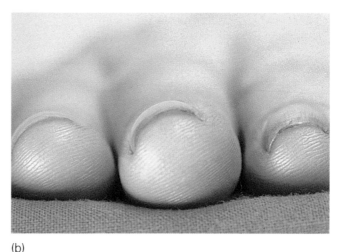

(b)

Figure 2.20
(a) Transverse curvature of nail; (b) transverse curvature of nail in yellow nail syndrome (before colour change).

(a)

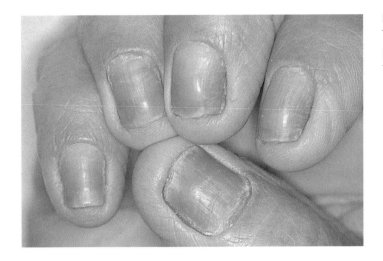

Figure 2.21
Transverse overcurvature in the pseudo yellow nail syndrome due to insecticide and weed killer.

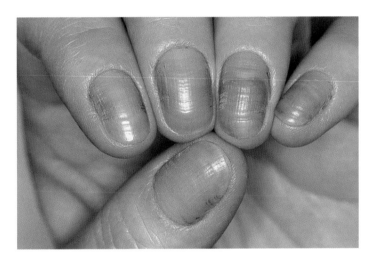

Figure 2.22
Transverse overcurvature in the yellow nail syndrome.

developmental abnormality which may be an autosomal dominant trait. The pathogenesis of the nail plate deformation has recently been clarified: the great toe nail, which is normally curved transversely, spreads around almost 40% of the dorsal aspect of the base of the terminal phalanx. Radiographs demonstrate that in people with pincer nails the base of the terminal phalanx is widened by lateral osteophytes that are even more pronounced on the medial aspect of the phalanx. By widening the transverse curvature of the nail at its proximal end it becomes more curved distally. This can easily be shown by trying to flatten a curved elastic sheet at one end: the other end will increase its curve. The asymmetry of the lateral osteophytes explains why the lateral deviation of the nail is even more pronounced than that of the distal phalanx.

Acquired pincer nails can be attributed to wearing ill-fitting shoes. These nails are not usually symmetrical and the lesser toe nails are not generally affected.

2

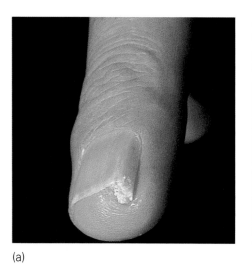

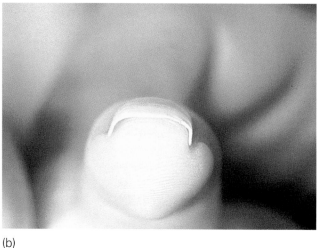

(a)   (b)

Figure 2.23
(a) Transverse overcurvature of nail: unilateral plicature; (b) transverse overcurvature of nail: bilateral plicatured variety (see Figure 2.17).

3   Underlying disease, such as subungual exostosis of the toes and inflammatory osteoarthritis, should always be looked for, especially if the fingers are involved.
4   Some dermatological disorders, especially psoriasis, may also cause transverse overcurvature of the nails.
5   Localized overcurvature is observed in onychomatricoma.

Tile-shaped nail

The tile-shaped nail presents with an increase in the transverse curvature; the lateral edges of the nail remain parallel.

Plicatured nail

In the plicatured nail the surface of the nail plate is almost flat, with one or both lateral margins being sharply angled forming vertical sides which are parallel (Figure 2.23). Although these

deformities may be associated with ingrowing nails, inflammatory oedema due to the constriction of the enclosed soft tissues is unusual.

DOLICHONYCHIA (LONG NAILS)

In dolichonychia the length of the nail is much greater than the width (Figure 2.24). It has been described in:

1   Ehlers–Danlos syndrome
2   Marfan's syndrome (Figure 2.25)
3   Eunuchoidism
4   Hypopituitarism
5   Hypohidrotic ectodermal dysplasia.

BRACHYONYCHIA (SHORT NAILS)

In brachyonychia (Figures 2.26–2.34) the width of the nail plate (and the nail bed) is

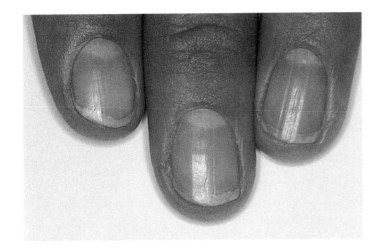

Figure 2.24
Dolichonychia (long nails).

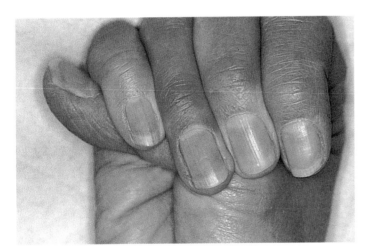

Figure 2.25
Dolichonychia in Marfan's
syndrome.

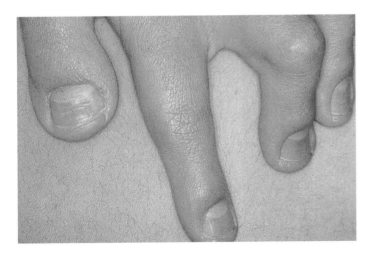

Figure 2.26
Brachyonychia: Rubinstein–Taybi
type, broad thumb. (Courtesy of
P. Souteyrand.)

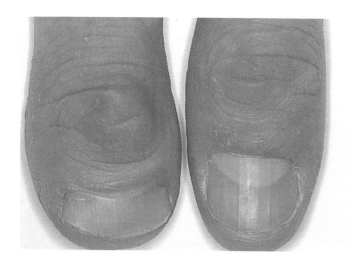

Figure 2.27
Brachyonychia (short nails).

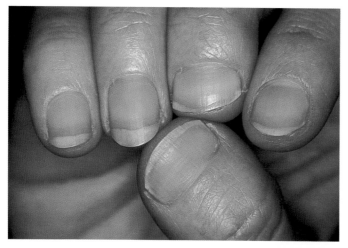

Figure 2.28
Brachyonychia of the thumb and
middle finger.

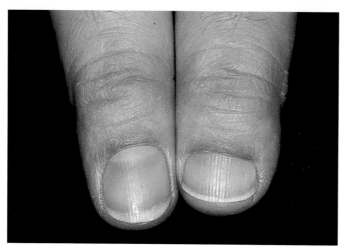

Figure 2.29
Brachyonychia – racquet nail of
one thumb.

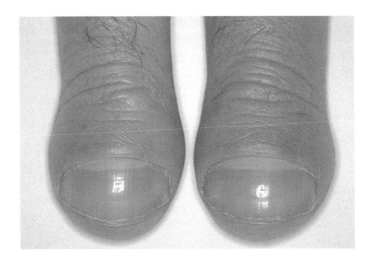

Figure 2.30
Bilateral brachyonychia – racquet nail associated with clubbing. (Courtesy of F. Daniel, Paris.)

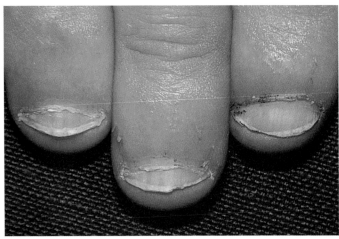

Figure 2.31
Brachyonychia – severe variant.

greater than the length. It may occur in isolation or in association with shortening of the terminal phalanx. This 'racquet thumb' is usually inherited as an autosomal dominant trait. All the fingers may rarely be involved. The epiphyses of the terminal phalanx of the thumb usually undergo closure between 13 and 14 years of age in girls, slightly later in boys. In individuals with this hereditary defect the epiphyseal line is obliterated on the affected side by 7–10 years of age, only occurring at the usual later age in the normal thumb. Since periosteal growth continues, the result is a deformed, racquet-like thumb.

Racquet nails have been reported in association with brachydactyly and multiple malignant Spiegler tumours. A syndrome of broad thumbs, broad great toes, facial abnormalities and mental retardation has also been described. Table 2.4 lists many well-recognized causes of short nails, while Table 2.5 gives details of the rarer hereditary and congenital conditions in which it can occur.

Table 2.4 Causes of brachyonychia

Congenital

Rubenstein–Taybi: 'broad thumbs' syndrome (Figure 2.26)

Micronychia with trisomy 21

Congenital malalignment – great toe nails

Acquired

Isolated defect: racquet thumb (Figures 2.27, 2.30, 2.31) (hereditary)

Nail biters (Figure 2.32)

Associated with bone resorption in hyperparathyroidism (Figure 2.33)

Psoriatic arthropathy (Figure 2.34)

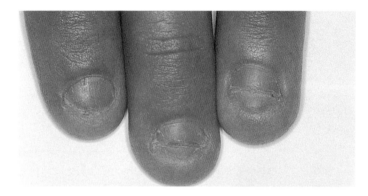

Figure 2.32
Brachyonychia – nail biting.

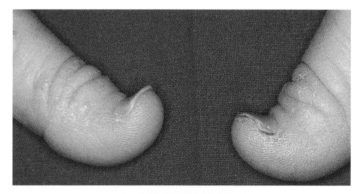

(a)

Figure 2.33
(a) Brachyonychia associated with bone resorption in hyperparathyroidism; (b) radiograph of (a). (Courtesy of B. Schubert.)

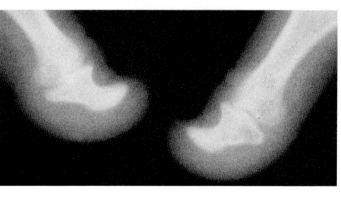

(b)

Table 2.5 Hereditary forms of broad nails (some also with pseudoclubbing)

Disease	Inheritance	Clinical features
Acrocephalosyndactyly	AD	Craniosynostosis, syndactyly, ankylosis and other skeletal deformities
Acrodysostosis	AD	Finger nails short, broad and oval in shape; short fingers; nasal and midface hypoplasia; mental retardation; growth failure; pigmented naevi
Berk-Tabatznik syndrome	?	Stub thumb, short terminal phalanges of all fingers except little finger; bilateral optic atrophy, cervical kyphosis
Familial mandibuloacral dysplasia	AR	Club-shaped terminal phalanges; mandibular hypoplasia, delayed cranial closure; dysplastic clavicles; atrophy of skin over hands and feet; alopecia
Keipert syndrome	AR or XR	Unusual facies with large nose; protruding upper lip; short and broad distal phalanges of halluces and fingers, except little finger
Larsen's syndrome	AR or AD	Stub thumbs, cylindrical fingers; flattened peculiar facies, wide-spaced eyes; multiple dislocations, short metacarpals
Nanocephalic dwarfism	AR	Low birthweight with adult head circumference; mental retardation; beak-like protrusion of nose; multiple osseous anomalies; clubbing of fingers
Otopalatodigital syndrome	XR or AR	Broad, short nails, especially of thumbs and great toes; mental retardation; prominent occiput; hypoplasia of facial bones; cloven palate; conductive deafness
Pleonosteosis	?	Short stature; spade-like thumbs with thick palmar pads; massive, 'knobby' thumbs; short, flexed fingers; limited joint motion with contractures
Pseudohypoparathyroidism	XD or AR	Short stature; round face; depressed nasal bridge; short metacarpals; mental retardation; cataracts in 25%; enamel hypoplasia; calcifications in skin
Puretic syndrome	?	Osteolysis of peripheral phalanges; stunted growth; contracture of joints; multiple subcutaneous nodules; atrophic sclerodermic skin
Rubinstein–Taybi syndrome	AD	Broad thumb with radial angulation and great toes; high palate; short stature; mental retardation; peculiar facies
Spiegler tumours and racquet nails	?	Brachydactyly; Turban tumours
Stub thumb with racquet nail (Figures 2.27, 2.30)	AD	No other defects; appears at the age of 7–10 years with early obliteration of the epiphyseal line

AD, autosomal dominant; AR, autosomal recessive; XD, sex-linked dominant; XR, sex-linked recessive

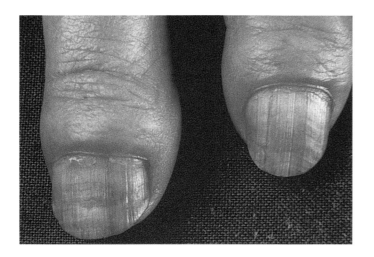

Figure 2.34
Brachyonychia in psoriatic arthropathy. (Courtesy of P. Combemale, Lyon.)

PARROT-BEAK NAILS

In this symmetrical overcurvature of the free edge, some finger nails mimic the beak of a parrot (Figures 2.35, 2.36); this shape disappears temporarily if the nails are soaked in lukewarm water for about 30 minutes. This condition is often not seen in clinical practice because such patients usually trim their nails close to the line of separation from the nail bed. Parrot-beak nails are a typical sign of severe acrosclerosis with distal phalangeal resorption. The nail plate bends around the shortened fingertip.

ROUND FINGERPAD

The round fingerpad sign describes a modification in the contour of the fingerpad, which changes from peaked to hemispheric. The sign is more common on the ring finger of patients with scleroderma or Raynaud's phenomenon (Figure 2.37).

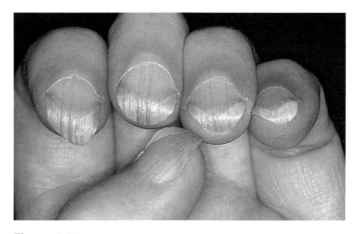

Figure 2.35
Parrot-beak nails.

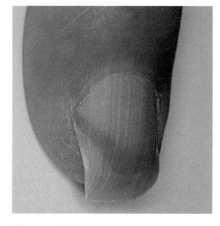

Figure 2.36
Parrot-beak nails – lateral view.

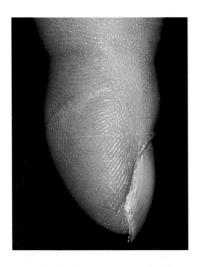

Figure 2.37
Fingerpad sign in scleroderma.

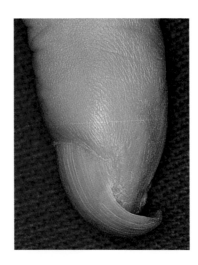

Figure 2.38
Claw-like nail.

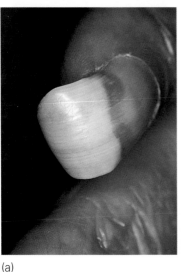

(a)

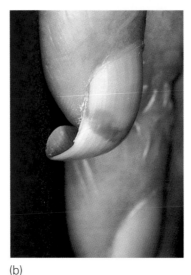

(b)

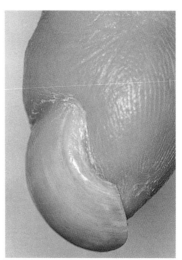

Figure 2.40
Hook nail.

Figure 2.39
(a, b) Claw-like nail – frontal and lateral views.

HOOK AND CLAW-LIKE NAILS

One or both little toe nails are often rounded like a claw. This condition predominates in women wearing high heels and narrow shoes and is often associated with the development of hyperkeratosis such as calluses on the feet. Congenital claw-like fingers and toe nails have been reported (Figures 2.38, 2.39). Claw nails may be curved dorsally showing a concave upper surface, resembling onychogryphosis or post-traumatic hook nail. In the nail–patella syndrome when the pointed lunula sign occurs, if the nail is not manicured it will tend to grow with a pointed tip, resembling a claw. Hook nails (Figure 2.40) may be an isolated defect, congenital or acquired (e.g. traumatic).

MICRONYCHIA, MACRONYCHIA AND POLYDACTYLY

In Iso–Kikuchi syndrome (congenital onychodysplasia of index finger nails, COIF) there are two types of micronychia. The most frequent is medially sited; in 'rolled' micronychia the nail is centrally located (Figures 2.41–2.45). Figures 2.46–2.48 illustrate other examples of congenital micronychia. Overlapping of the nail surface by an enlarged lateral nail fold may result in apparent micronychia (Turner's syndrome).

In macronychia the nails of one or more digits are wider than normal, with nail bed and

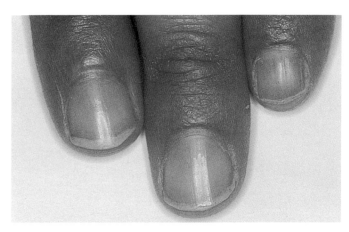

Figure 2.41
Micronychia involving one finger.

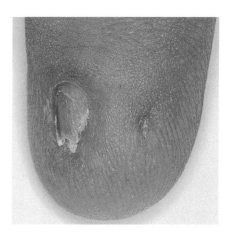

Figure 2.42
Micronychia – congenital onychodysplasia of index finger nails (COIF) syndrome.

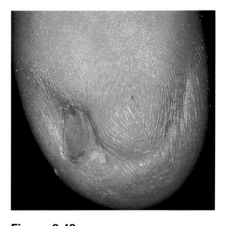

Figure 2.43
Micronychia in COIF syndrome.

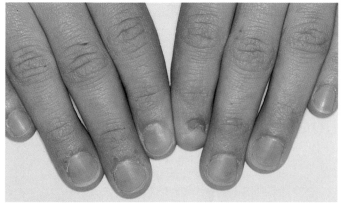

Figure 2.44
Rolled micronychia in COIF syndrome.

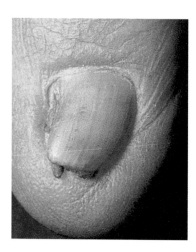

Figure 2.45
Rolled micronychia.

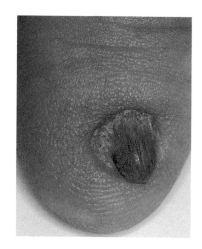

Figure 2.46
Micronychia in congenital ectodermal dysplasia.

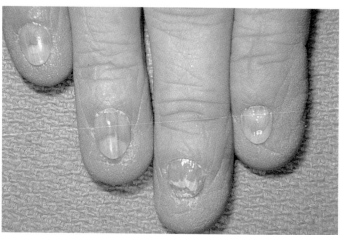

Figure 2.47
Micronychia – 'small nail field' defect in hidrotic ectodermal dysplasia. (Courtesy of L. Norton.)

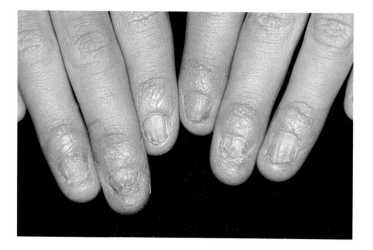

Figure 2.48
Micronychia in a child affected by AEC syndrome (ankyloblepharon, ectodermal dysplasia and cleft palate).

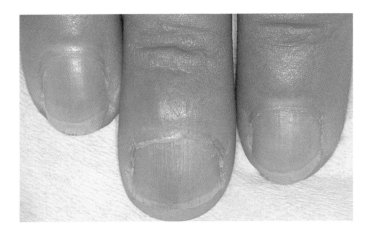

Figure 2.49
Macronychia of the middle finger.

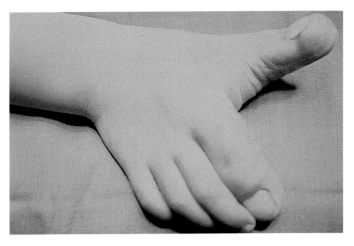

Figure 2.50
Macronychia with macrodactyly in
Proteus syndrome.

Table 2.6 Causes of micronychia and macronychia

Congenital	Acquired
Ectodermal dysplasias (Figures 2.46, 2.47)	Fetal teratogens
Congenital onchodysplasia of index finger	hydantoinates
nails (Figures 2.42–2.44)	alcohol
Bifid toe (Figure 2.51)	warfarin
Dyskeratosis congenita	Amniotic bands
Chromosomal abnormalities	
Nail–patella syndrome	

matrix similarly affected (Figure 2.49). This may
occur as an isolated defect or in association
with megadactyly, as in von Recklinghausen's disease, epiloia and Proteus syndrome (Figure
2.50). Table 2.6 lists the known associations of
micronychia and macronychia.

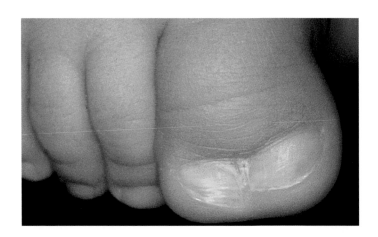

Figure 2.51
Bifid toe.

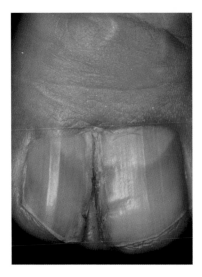

Figure 2.52
Bifid thumb.

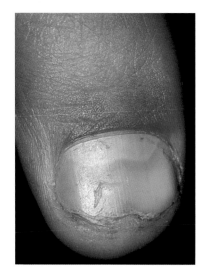

Figure 2.53
Bifid lunula
in a child
with
congenital
polydactyly.

Duplication of the thumb is a sign of congenital polydactyly, one of the most common anomalies of the hand. The frequency of polydactyly of the hands has been estimated to be 0.37%; it is more common than polydactyly of the feet (Figure 2.51). Seven types of thumb polydactyly can be distinguished according to the level of bone bifurcation. Patients with types 1 and 2 thumb polydactyly have two distinct nails separated by a longitudinal incision or a unique nail with a central indentation of the distal margin (Figures 2.52, 2.53). Symphalangism is commonly observed. Thumb polydactyly may be sporadic, usually transmitted as an autosomal dominant trait with variable expressivity. A similar clinical picture can be seen in the great toe with bifurcation of the terminal phalanx and duplication of the nail. Early treatment is important to maximize functional restoration and aesthetic results.

> **A bifid lunula can also be a sign of polydactyly**

WORN-DOWN, SHINY NAILS

Patients with atopic dermatitis or chronic erythroderma may be 'chronic scratchers and rubbers'. The surface of the nail plate becomes glossy and shiny and the free edge is worn away (Figures 2.54, 2.55). This condition, also called *usure des ongles*, may also occur in many different manual occupations. It has recently been described as a particular hazard of individuals handling heavy plastic bags.

The term 'bidet nails' describes an unusual nail configuration abnormality characterized by thinning and excavation of the central portion of the distal nail plate in a triangular pattern

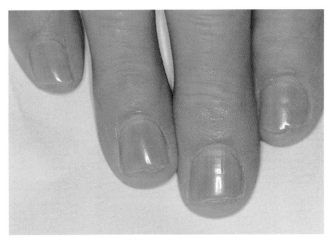

Figure 2.54
Worn-down, shiny nails (*usure des ongles*), due to chronic rubbing and scratching.

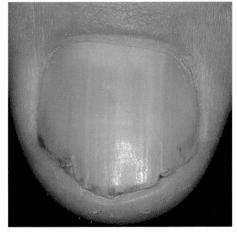

Figure 2.55
Darier's disease – worn-down tips due to intrinsic keratinization defect; note associated white lines.

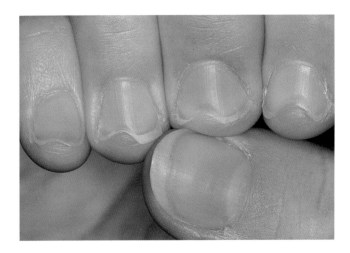

Figure 2.56
Bidet nails.

Shiny finger nails usually imply severe scratching or rubbing of the skin

with distal base (Figure 2.56). The distal margin shows a V-shaped incisure. 'Bidet nails' result from chronic rubbing of the nails against a hard surface and typically affect the middle three fingers of the dominant hand.

The following conditions may be responsible:

- worn-down nails: occupational causes
- smooth, shiny nails: atopic eczema; pruritic lymphoma; chronic pruritus
- distal fraying: trauma; Darier's disease (Figure 2.55); old age; nail scratching.

ANONYCHIA AND ONYCHATROPHY

It is impossible to differentiate completely between anonychia and onychatrophy in the light of current knowledge. In principle the term 'anonychia' (total or partial) is probably best reserved for conditions in which the nail has failed to develop; 'onychatrophy' should be used to describe processes in which the nail has initially formed satisfactorily and then shown total or partial regression. Table 2.7 lists the causes of anonychia and onychatrophy.

In aplastic anonychia, a rare congenital disorder occasionally associated with other defects such as ectrodactyly, the nail never forms. Loose, horny masses are produced by the metaplastic squamous epithelium of the matrix and the nail bed in anonychia keratodes. Hypoplasia of the nail plates is a hallmark of the nail–patella syndrome; in the least affected cases only the ulnar half of each thumb nail is missing.

Table 2.7 Causes of anonychia and onychatrophy

Permanent hypo- or anonychia (Figures 2.57–2.60)
+/– ectrodactyly
+/– dental malformations
Nail–patella syndrome (Figure 2.60)
Congenital onychodysplasia of index finger
Coffin–Siris syndrome with many congenital defects
DOOR syndrome (deafness, onychodystrophy, osteodystrophy, mental retardation) (Figure 2.58)

Onychatrophy (Figures 2.61–2.78)
With pterygium (Figure 2.71)
lichen planus (Figures 2.71, 2.72)
acrosclerosis (Figure 2.63)
onychotillomania (Figures 2.76, 2.77)
Lesch–Nyhan syndrome
chronic graft-versus-host disease
Stevens–Johnson or Lyell's syndrome (Figure 2.66)
cicatricial pemphigoid (Figure 2.64)
Without pterygium
severe paronychia with nail dystrophy
Stevens–Johnson or Lyell's syndrome (Figure 2.66)
epidermolysis bullosa (Figures 2.67–2.69)
amyloidosis
etretinate nail dystrophy (Figure 2.62)
idiopathic atrophy of childhood (Figure 2.75)
severe psoriatic nail dystrophy (Figure 2.70)

Onychatrophy presents as a reduction in size and thickness of the nail plate, often accompanied by fragmentation and splitting, for example in lichen planus. It may progressively worsen, scar tissue eventually replacing the atrophic nail plate.

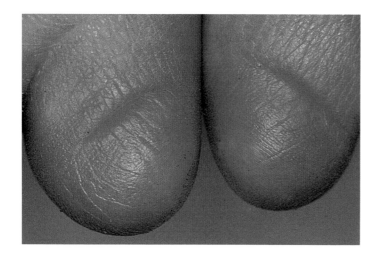

Figure 2.57
Congenital absence of nails.

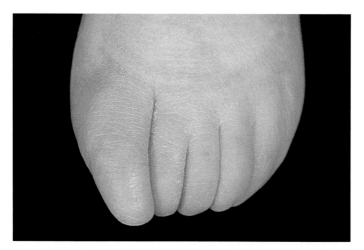

Figure 2.58
Congenital absence of nails in the
DOOR syndrome. (Courtesy of
Professor Nevin, Belfast.)

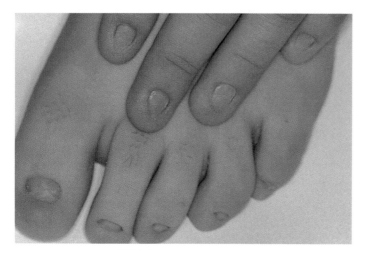

Figure 2.59
Micronychia in congenital
ectodermal dysplasia.

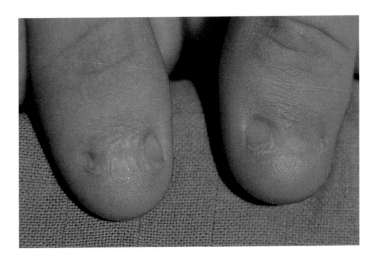

Figure 2.60
Partial anonychia in the nail–patella syndrome.

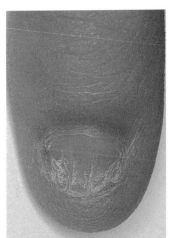

Figure 2.61
Onychatrophy – ectodermal dysplasia.

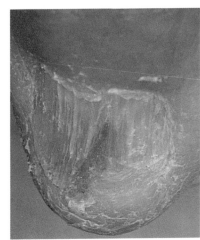

Figure 2.62
Onychatrophy due to oral etretinate therapy. (Courtesy of B. Kalis, Reims)

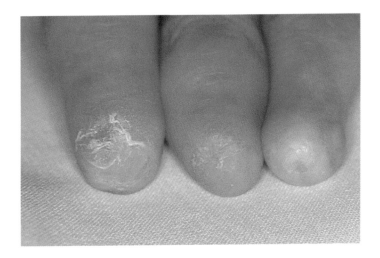

Figure 2.63
Onychatrophy – acrosclerosis.

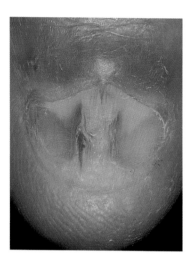

Figure 2.64
Onychatrophy
and
koilonychia in
cicatricial
pemphigoid.

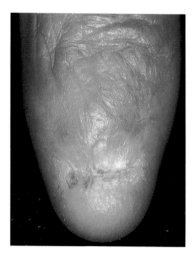

Figure 2.65
Onychatrophy
due to
sarcoidosis
with bone
involvement.

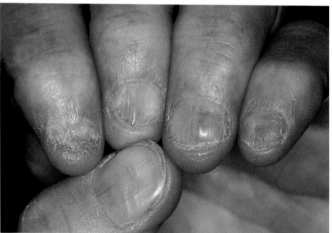

Figure 2.66
Onychatrophy after
Stevens–Johnson syndrome.

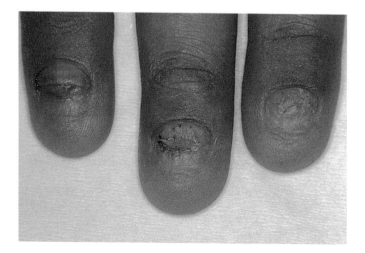

Figure 2.67
Onychatrophy in epidermolysis
bullosa.

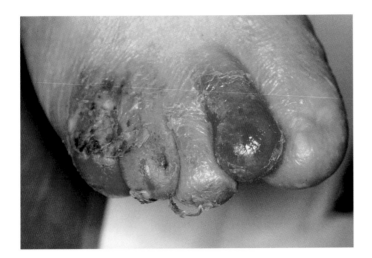

Figure 2.68
Onychatrophy in a child with epidermolysis bullosa dystrophica.

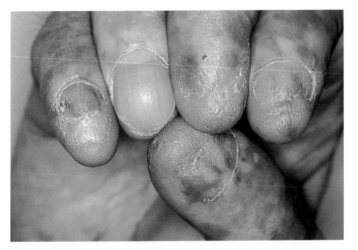

Figure 2.69
Onychatrophy – epidermolysis bullosa dystrophica.

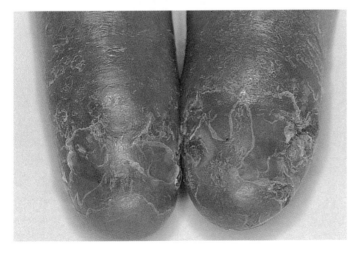

Figure 2.70
Onychatrophy – pustular psoriasis.

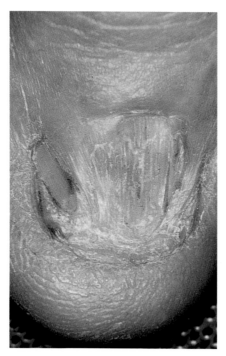

Figure 2.71
Onychatrophy – lichen planus.

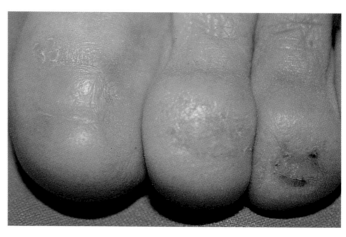

Figure 2.72
Onychatrophy – lichen planus with total nail loss.

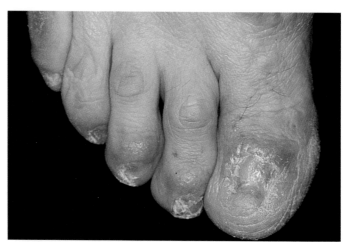

Figure 2.73
Severe onychatrophy.

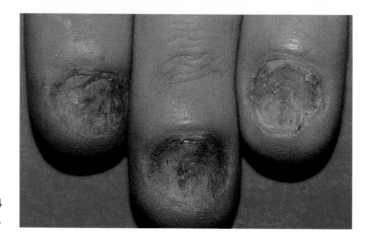

Figure 2.74
Onychatrophy – severe nail biting.

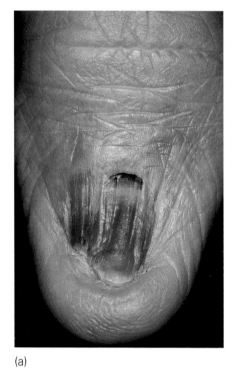

(a)

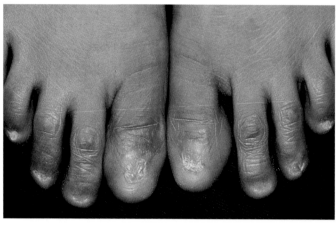

(b)

Figure 2.75
(a, b) Idiopathic atrophy of the nails: onychatrophy and
anonychia.

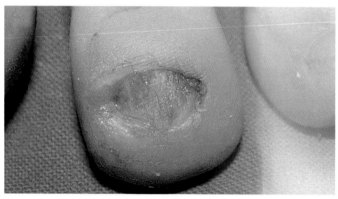

Figure 2.76
Onychatrophy – onychotillomania.

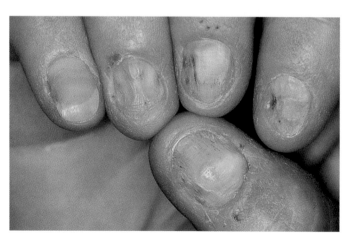

Figure 2.77
Onychatrophy – onychotillomania.

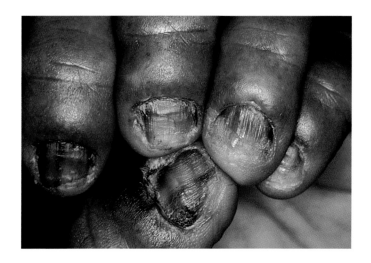

Figure 2.78
Onychotillomania – onychatrophy and pigmentation.

FURTHER READING

Clubbing

Dickinson CJ, Martin JF (1987) Megakaryocytes and platelet clumps as the cause of finger clubbing, *Lancet* **ii**: 1434–1435.

Fischer DS, Singer DH, Feldman SM (1964) Clubbing, a review, with emphasis on hereditary acropachy, *Medicine* **43**: 459–479.

Myers KA, Farquhar DRE (2001). Does this patient have clubbing? *JAMA* **286**: 341–347.

Koilonychia

Hogan GR, Jones B (1970) The relationship between koilonychia and iron deficiency in infants, *J Pediatr* **77**: 1054–1057.

Stone OJ (1985) Clubbing and koilonychia, *Dermatol Clin* **3**: 485–490.

Transverse overcurvature

Cohen P, Milewicz DM (1993) Dolichonychia in a patient with the Marfan syndrome, *J Dermatol* **20**: 779–782.

Cornelius CE, Shelley WB (1968) Pincer nail syndrome, *Arch Surg* **96**: 321–322.

Haneke E (1992) Etiopathogénie et traitement de l'hypercourbure transversale de l'ongle du gros orteil, *J Méd Esth Chir Dermatol* **19**: 123–127.

Brachyonychia

Rubinstein JH (1969) The broad thumbs syndrome progress report 1968, *Birth Defects: Original Article Series* **V(2)**: 25–41.

Round fingerpad sign

Mizutani H, Mizutani T, Okada H *et al* (1991) Round fingerpad sign: an early sign of scleroderma, *J Am Acad Dermatol* **24**: 67–69.

Micro- and macronychia

Kikuchi I (1985) Congenital polyonychias: reduction versus duplication digit malformations, *Int J Dermatol* **24**: 211–215.

Telfer NR, Barth JH, Dawber RPR (1988) Congenital and hereditary nail dystrophies: an embryological approach to classification, *Clin Exp Dermatol* **13**: 160–163.

Worn-down and shiny nails

Baran R, Moulin G (1999). The bidet nail: a French variant of the worn-down nail syndrome, *Br J Dermatol* **140**: 377.

Anonychia and nail atrophy

Zaias N (1970) The nail in lichen planus, *Arch Dermatol* **101**: 264–271.

Polydactyly

Tosti A, Paoluzzi P, Baran R (1992) Doubled nail of the thumb: a rare form of polydactyly, *Dermatology* **184**: 216–218.

3 Modifications of the nail surface

Antonella Tosti, Robert Baran, Rodney PR Dawber, Eckart Haneke

Longitudinal lines • Herringbone nails • Transverse lines • Pitting and rippling • Trachyonychia (rough nails) • Onychoschizia (lamellar splitting) • Further reading

LONGITUDINAL LINES

Longitudinal lines, or striations, may appear as indented grooves or projecting ridges (Figures 3.1–3.16).

> A single longitudinal nail fissure is most likely due to minor trauma

Longitudinal grooves

Longitudinal grooves represent long-lasting abnormalities and can develop under the following conditions:

1   Grooves with a physiological cause appear as shallow and delicate furrows, usually parallel, and separated by low, projecting ridges. They become more prominent with age and in certain pathological states, such as lichen planus, rheumatoid arthritis, peripheral vascular

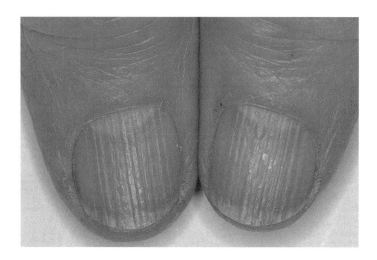

Figure 3.1
Longitudinal lines associated with old age.

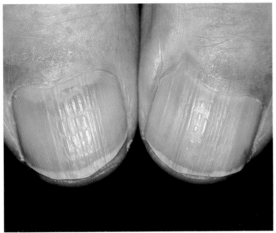

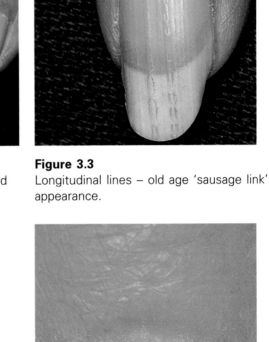

Figure 3.2
Longitudinal lines in a patient with rheumatoid arthritis.

Figure 3.3
Longitudinal lines – old age 'sausage link' appearance.

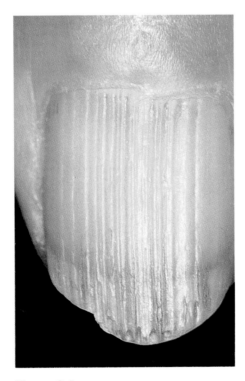

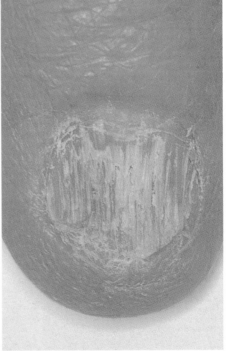

Figure 3.4
Longitudinal lines – prominent old age changes, which may occur earlier with chronic arterial impairment.

Figure 3.5
Longitudinal dystrophy in lichen planus.

(arterial) insufficiency, Darier's disease and other genetic abnormalities.

2 Onychorrhexis consists of a series of narrow, longitudinal, parallel superficial furrows with the appearance of having been scratched by an awl. Sometimes dust becomes ingrained into the nail surface. Splitting of the free edge is common. Onychorrhexis reflects severe nail matrix damage and is quite typical of nail lichen planus (Figures 3.6, 3.7). It is also observed in lichen striatus where it is

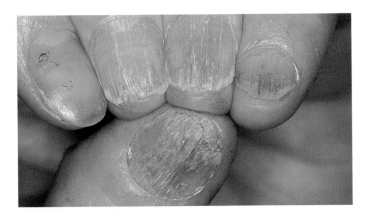

Figure 3.6
Mild onychorrhexis in lichen planus.

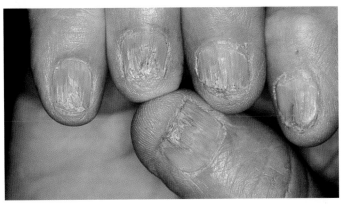

(a)

Figure 3.7
(a, b) Severe onychorrhexis and nail thinning in lichen planus.

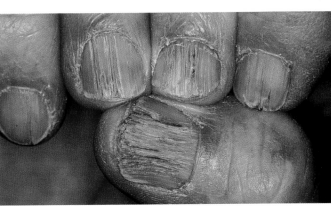

(b)

limited to a heminail. It may be an early sign of systemic amyloidosis; where it is often associated with splinter haemorrhages.

3 Tumours such as myxoid cysts and warts in the proximal nail fold area may exert pressure on the nail matrix and produce a wide, deep, longitudinal groove or canal,

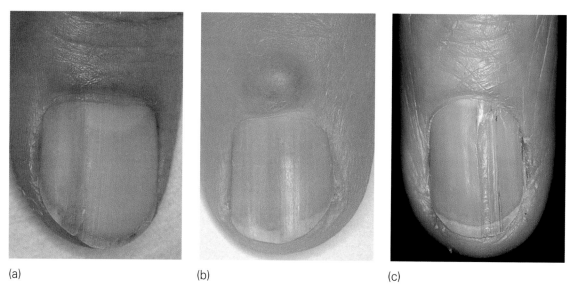

(a)   (b)   (c)

Figure 3.8
Longitudinal nail groove due to (a) glomus tumour, (b) myxoid cyst, (c) fibrokeratoma.

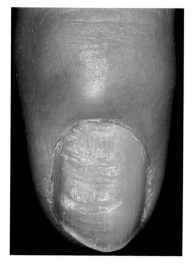
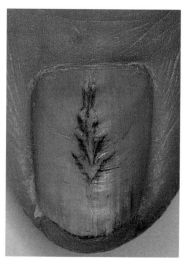
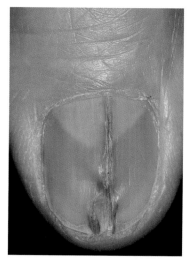

Figure 3.9
Myxoid cyst – longitudinal groove and Beau's lines.

Figure 3.10
Heller's median canaliform dystrophy (Leclercq's variant).

Figure 3.11
Heller's median canaliform dystrophy.

which disappears if the cause is removed (Figures 3.8, 3.9).

4 Median nail dystrophy (Figures 3.10, 3.11) is an uncommon condition consisting of a longitudinal defect of the thumb nails in the midline or just off-centre, starting at the cuticle and growing out of the free edge. It may be associated with an enlarged lunula. In early descriptions, the base of the 2–5 mm wide groove with steep edges showed numerous transverse defects. In some cases median longitudinal ridges have been observed, occasionally combined with fissures and/or a groove, developed from the distal edge of the nail plate to the matrix. Often a few short, feathery cracks, chevron-shaped, extend laterally from the split – the 'inverted fir tree' appearance. The so-called naevus striatus symmetricus of the thumbs corresponds to this form. Median nail dystrophy is usually symmetrical and most often affects the thumbs. Sometimes other fingers are involved, the toes less commonly (usually the great toe). After several months or years, the nail returns to normal but recurrences are not rare. Familial cases have been recorded. The aetiology is unknown, although it has been suggested that it is due to self-inflicted trauma resulting from a tic or habit (Figures 3.12, 3.13). Treatment of recalcitrant cases may be identical to that for post-traumatic nail splitting.

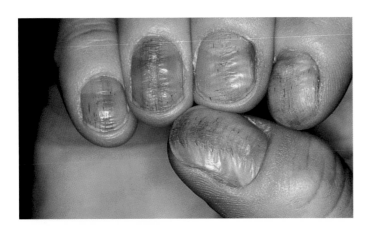

Figure 3.12
Onychotillomania – median nail dystrophy of several nails.

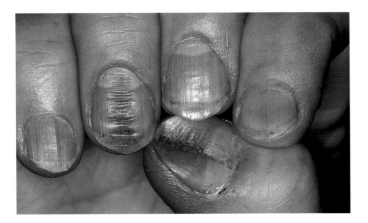

Figure 3.13
Onychotillomania – severe median nail dystrophy of the thumb and third finger nail.

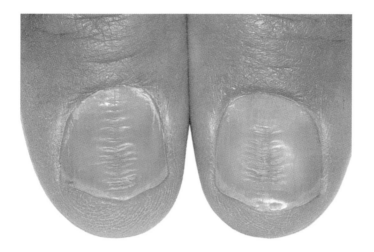

Figure 3.14
Central longitudinal grooved
dystrophy, self-induced by trauma
to the matrix.

5 A central longitudinal depression is found in 'washboard' nail plates, caused by chronic, mechanical injury (Figures 3.14–3.16). Unlike median nail dystrophy (Heller's dystrophy), the cuticle is pushed back and there is accompanying inflammation and/or thickening of the proximal nail fold. Splits due to trauma, or those occurring in the nail–patella syndrome and in pterygium, are usually obvious. Longitudinal splits may also result from Raynaud's disease, lichen striatus and trachyonychia. Nail wrapping (see Chapter 9) may lessen the disability produced by the fissure; the proximal nail fold must be protected from repeated minor trauma.

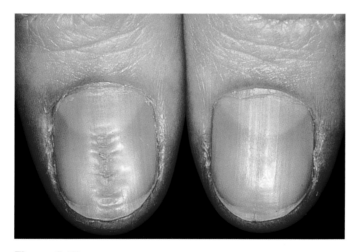

Figure 3.15
Unilateral central longitudinal grooved dystrophy.

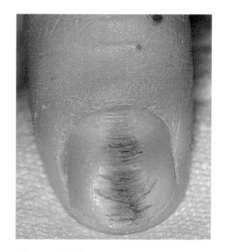

Figure 3.16
Deep groove plus transverse
lines – self-induced matrix
trauma.

Longitudinal ridges

Small rectilinear projections extend from the proximal nail fold as far as the free edge of the nail, or they may stop short. They may be interrupted at regular intervals, giving rise to a beaded appearance. Sometimes a wide, longitudinal median ridge has the appearance, in cross-section, of a circumflex accent. The condition is inherited and affects mainly the thumb and index fingers of both hands.

Table 3.1 shows the principal causes of longitudinal lines and grooves.

Table 3.1 Causes of longitudinal lines

Coloured lines

White	*See* leukonychia (pages 128–134)
Black	*See* melanonychia (pages 134–139)
Red	Darier's disease (*see* Figure 2.55)
	Vascular tumours
	Glomus (Figure 3.8)
	Cirsoid

Linear ridges

Single	Familial
	Median canaliform dystrophy (Figure 3.10)
	Trauma (isolated or repeated)
	Tumours
Multiple	Normal; increase with age after early adulthood (Figures 3.1, 3.3, 3.4)
	With all causes of thin nail plates
	Lichen planus (Figure 3.5)
	Rheumatoid arthritis
	Graft-versus-host disease
	Psoriasis
	Darier's disease
	Poor circulation
	Collagen vascular diseases
	Radiation
	Frostbite
	Alopecia areata
	Nail–patella syndrome
	Systemic amyloidosis

HERRINGBONE NAILS

The pattern of nail ridging known as 'herringbone nails', with oblique lines pointing centrally to meet in the midline, has been reported as an uncommon phenomenon occurring in childhood (Figure 3.17). It characteristically disappears as the child grows. Less obvious, similar lines may be seen associated with the pointed matrix of the nail–patella syndrome.

TRANSVERSE LINES

Transverse, band-like depressions extending from one lateral edge of the nail to the other, and affecting all nails at corresponding levels, are called Beau's lines (Figures 3.18–3.22). They may be noted after any severe, sudden (particularly febrile) illness. In milder cases the nails of the thumb and the great toe are the most reliable markers, as the former supplies information for the previous 6–9 months and the latter shows evidence of disease for up to 2 years (relating to the different rates of linear nail growth).

The width of the transverse groove relates to the duration of the disease that has affected the matrix. The distal limit of the furrow, if abrupt, indicates a sudden attack of disease; if sloping, a more protracted onset. The proximal limit of the depression may be abrupt, and both limits may well be sloped. If the the disease can completely inhibit the activity of the matrix for 1–2 weeks or longer, the transverse depression will result in total division of the nail plate, a defect known as 'onychomadesis' (Figures 3.23, 3.24). As the nail adheres firmly to the nail bed the onychomadesis remains latent for several weeks before leading to temporary shedding.

> **The presence of Beau's lines on all 20 nails is usually the result of systemic disease**

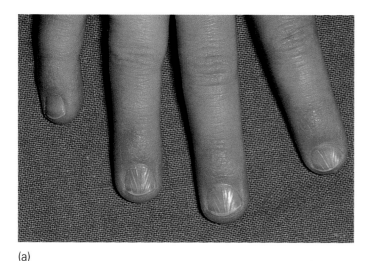

(a)

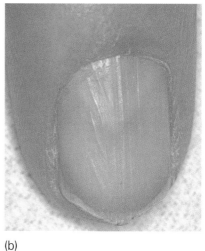

(b)

Figure 3.17
(a) Herringbone nail appearance with oblique lines meeting in the midline – a temporary change of early childhood; (b) nail–patella syndrome – more subtle, but similar lines to (a); associated with pointed lunula. (Part (a) from Parry EJ, Morley WN, Dawber RPR (1995), Herringbone nails: an uncommon variant of nail growth in childhood? *Br J Dermatol* **132**: 1021–1022.)

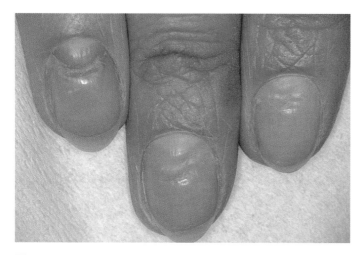

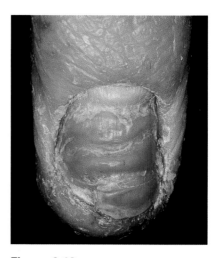

Figure 3.18
Beau's lines.

Figure 3.19
Beau's lines – contact dermatitis.

Transverse furrows may be due to measles in childhood, zinc deficiency (often multiple), Stevens–Johnson and Lyell's syndromes, cytotoxic drugs and many other non-specific events. Beau's lines can also be physiological, e.g. marks appearing with each menstrual cycle, particularly in dysmenorrhoea. They have also been noted in babies aged 4–5

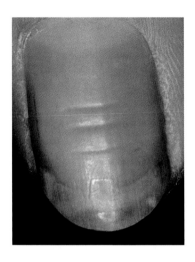

Figure 3.20
Transverse lines due to chemotherapy cycles. (Courtesy of L. Requena.)

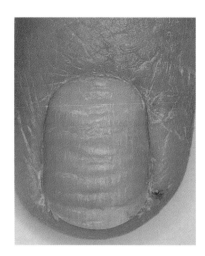

Figure 3.21
Beau's lines in psoriasis.

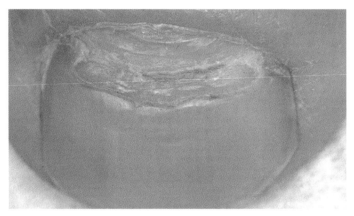

Figure 3.22
Long Beau's line (depression) due to more prolonged arrest of growth. (Courtesy of J. P. Ortonne, Nice.)

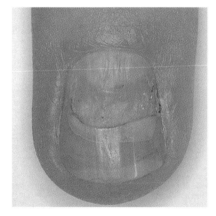

Figure 3.23
Onychomadesis due to bleomycin therapy for warts on the proximal nail fold.

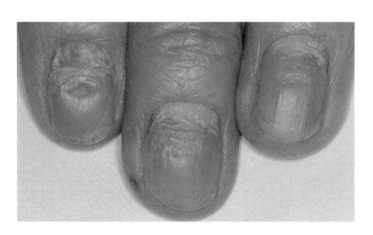

Figure 3.24
Beau's lines and onychomadesis due to psoriasis.

Table 3.2 Causes of transverse grooves

Common
   High fever
   Postnatal
   Menstrual cycle (multiple grooves),
      dysmenorrhoea
   Measles
   Trauma
   Chronic paronychia
   Local inflammation
   Chronic eczema

Uncommon
   Kawasaki syndrome
   Stevens–Johnson syndrome
   Cytotoxic drugs
   Acrodermatitis enteropathica and zinc
      deficiency
   Hypoparathyroidism
   Syphilis
   Mouth, hand and foot disease
   Radiation
   Carpal tunnel syndrome

weeks, without any obvious cause. When only a few digits are involved this may indicate trauma, carpal tunnel syndrome, chronic paronychia or chronic eczema. If the lines appear following a chronic condition, they are often numerous and curvilinear.

When a series of transverse grooves parallels the proximal nail fold the cause is likely to be repeated trauma from overzealous manicuring. 'Rhythmic' parallel transverse grooves may be an isolated sign of psoriasis, equivalent to patterned pitting.

The nervous habit of pushing back the cuticle usually affects the thumbs which are damaged by either the thumb nail of the opposite hand or the index finger nail of the corresponding hand: symmetrical involvement of the thumbs is the rule and damage is most commonly effected by the thumb nail of the

other hand (see Figures 3.14, 3.16). Occasionally only one thumb is affected; rarely, other digits may be involved, the thumb reversing roles and creating the damage. This produces:

1 Swelling, redness and scaling of the proximal nail fold from the mechanical injury.
2 Multiple horizontal grooves that do not extend to the lateral margin of the nail; often filled with debris, they are interspersed between the ridges.
3 A large central longitudinal or slightly lateral depression along the nail mimicking median canaliform dystrophy, with an enlarged lunula.

Table 3.2 lists causes of transverse groove formation.

PITTING AND RIPPLING

Pitting and rippling are also known as pits, onychia punctata, erosions and Rosenau's depressions. Pits develop as a result of defective nail formation in punctate areas located in the proximal portion of the nail matrix. The surface of the nail plate is studded with small punctate depressions which vary in number, size, depth and shape. The depth and width of the pits relates to the extent of the matrix involved; their length is determined by the duration of the matrix damage. Pits result from a defective keratinization of the proximal matrix with persistence of parakeratotic cells in the nail plate surface. These cells are easily shed, leaving the punctate depression (Figure 3.25). They may be randomly distributed or uniformly arranged in series along one or several longitudinal lines; they are sometimes arranged in a criss-cross pattern and may resemble the external surface of a thimble.

It has been shown that regular pitting may convert to rippling or ridging, and these two conditions appear, at times, to be variants of

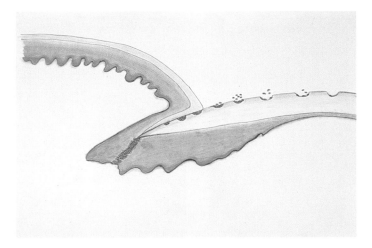

Figure 3.25
Pit formation.

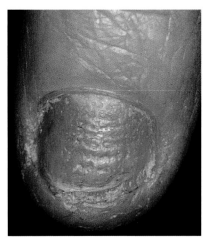

Figure 3.26
Multiple nail pits, arranged in transverse lines.

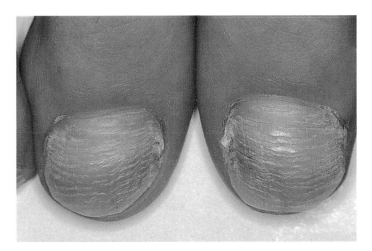

Figure 3.27
Multiple nail pits – similar to Figure 3.26, but more lined in appearance.

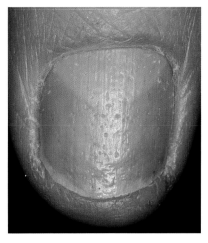

Figure 3.28
Pits in the proximal nail plate are still covered by parakeratotic scales.

uniform pitting (Figures 3.26–3.28). Nails showing diffuse pitting grow faster than the apparently normal nails in psoriasis. Occasional pits occur on normal nails. Deep pits can be attributed to psoriasis, and profuse pitting is most often due to this condition (Figures 3.29, 3.30). In alopecia areata (Figure 3.31) shallow pits are usually seen and they are often numerous, leading to trachyonychia (rough nail) and twenty-nail dystrophy; however, curiously, one nail often remains unaffected for a long time. Pits may also occur in eczema or occupational

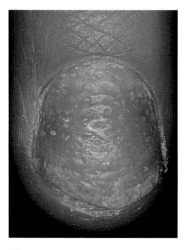

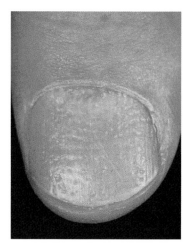

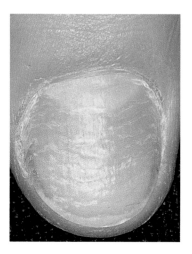

Figure 3.29
Multiple nail pits due to psoriasis.

Figure 3.30
Diffuse pitting of the whole nail in psoriasis.

Figure 3.31
Multiple nail pits – 'rippled' effect in alopecia areata.

Table 3.3 Causes of pitting

Common
  Psoriasis (Figures 3.26, 3.27, 3.29, 3.30)
  Alopecia areata (Figure 3.31)
  Eczema
  Occupational trauma
  Parakeratosis pustulosa

Uncommon
  Normal
  Pityriasis rosea
  Secondary syphilis
  Sarcoidosis
  Reiter's syndrome
  Lichen planus

Large, deep and irregular pits are common in psoriasis and eczema
Small, superficial and regular pits are typical of alopecia areata
An isolated pit is not diagnostic and may be due to minor trauma

trauma. In some cases a genetic basis is thought likely. In secondary syphilis and pityriasis rosea pitting occurs rarely. One case of the latter has been observed with the pits distributed on all the finger nails at corresponding levels, analogous to Beau's lines.

Table 3.3 lists the causes of nail pitting.

TRACHYONYCHIA (ROUGH NAILS)

The term 'twenty-nail dystrophy' or trachyonychia describes a spectrum of nail plate surface abnormalities that result in nail roughness (Figures 3.32–3.38). Patients with trachyonychia can be divided into two main groups:

1 Trachyonychia and a past history or clinical evidence of alopecia areata.
2 Isolated nail involvement (idiopathic trachyonychia).

Twenty-nail dystrophy usually occurs sporadically but a few familial and hereditary cases

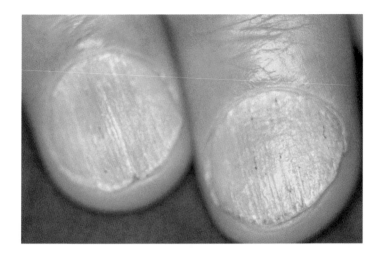

Figure 3.32
Trachyonychia (rough nails) due to
alopecia areata.

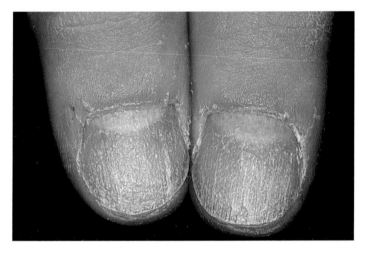

Figure 3.33
Trachyonychia – shiny variety.

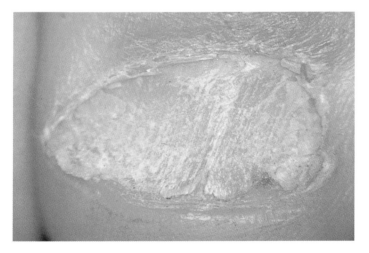

Figure 3.34
Trachyonychia – idiopathic.

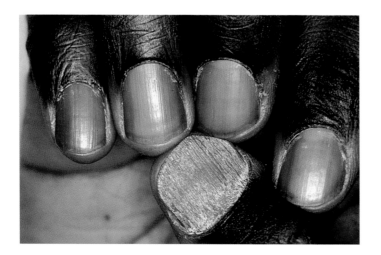

Figure 3.35
Trachyonychia – involvement of a single nail.

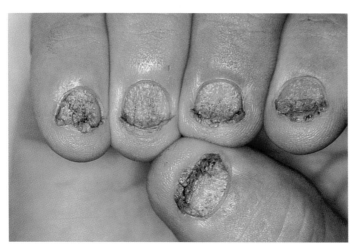

Figure 3.36
Trachyonychia in a manual worker.

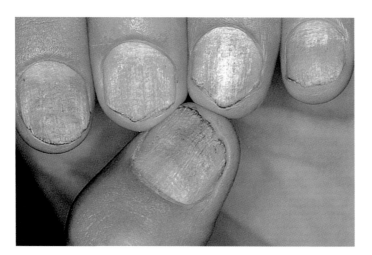

Figure 3.37
Trachyonychia – lichen planus.

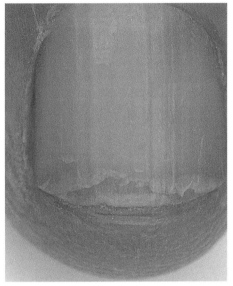

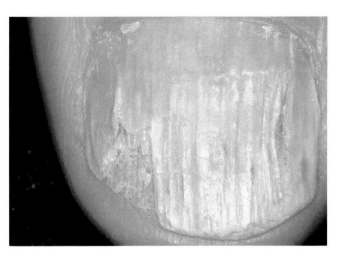

Figure 3.41
Onychoschizia and onychorrhexis due to lichen planus.

Figure 3.39
Onychoschizia (lamellar splitting or layering).

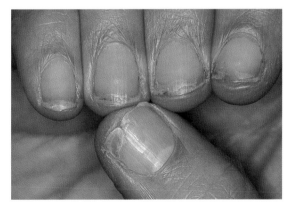

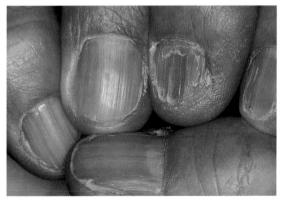

Figure 3.40
Onychoschizia lamellina affecting several finger nails.

Figure 3.42
Onychoschizia and onychorrhexis due to systemic amyloidosis.

dominant chondrodysplasia punctata and in polycythaemia vera. It may be seen in the proximal portion of the nail in lichen planus (Figure 3.41), and also as a result of oral retinoid therapy (Figures 3.43, 3.44).

The term 'elkonyxis' indicates proximal onychoschizia that is especially seen in patients taking oral retinoids.

Table 3.5 lists the known causes of onychoschizia.

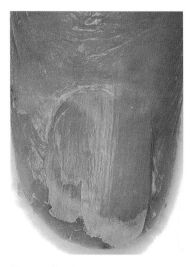

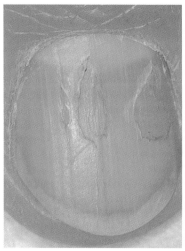

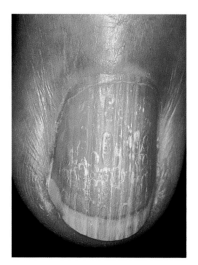

Figure 3.43
Onychoschizia due to oral
retinoid therapy.

Figure 3.44
Proximal onychoschizia due to
oral retinoid therapy.

Figure 3.45
Superficial nail fragility due to
nail lacquer.

Table 3.5 Causes of onychoschizia (lamellar splitting)

Proximal	**Distal**
Psoriasis	Chemical injury
Lichen planus (Figure 3.41)	Old age
Retinoid therapy (Figure 3.43)	Repeated wetting
	Chondrodysplasia punctata of the nails (X-linked)
	Polycythaemia vera

FURTHER READING

Herringbone nails

Parry EJ, Morley WN, Dawber RPR (1995) Herringbone nails: an uncommon variant of nail growth in childhood? *Br J Dermatol* **132**: 1021–1022.

Trachyonychia

Baran R, Dawber RPR (1987) Twenty nail dystrophy of childhood: a misnamed syndrome, *Cutis* **39**: 481–482.

Tosti A, Fanti PA, Morelli R, Bardazzi F (1991) Trachyonychia associated with alopecia areata: a clinical and pathological study, *J Am Acad Dermatol* **25**: 266–270.

Tosti A, Bardazzi F, Piraccini BM, Fanti PA (1994) Trachyonychia (twenty nail dystrophy): clinical and pathological study of 23 patients, *Br J Dermatol* **131**: 866–872.

Onychoschizia

Shelley WB, Shelley ED (1984) Onychoschizia: scanning electron microscopy, *J Am Acad Dermatol* **10**: 623–627.

4 Nail plate and soft tissue abnormalities

Robert Baran, Rodney PR Dawber, Eckart Haneke, Antonella Tosti

Onycholysis • Onychomadesis and shedding • Hypertrophic nail and subungual hyperkeratosis • Splinter haemorrhages and haematomas • Dorsal and ventral pterygium • Further reading

ONYCHOLYSIS

Onycholysis refers to the detachment of the nail from its bed at its distal and/or lateral attachments (Figure 4.1).

The pattern of separation of the plate from the nail bed takes many forms. Sometimes it resembles closely the damage from a splinter under the nail, the detachment extending proximally along a convex line, giving the appearance of a half-moon. When the process reaches the matrix, onycholysis becomes complete. Involvement of the lateral edge of the nail plate alone is less common. In certain cases the free edge rises up like a hood, or coils upon itself like a roll of paper. Onycholysis creates a subungual space which gathers dirt and keratinous debris; the greyish-white colour is due to the presence of air under the nail but the colour may vary from yellow to brown, depending on the aetiology. This area is sometimes malodorous.

In psoriasis (Figures 4.2–4.4) there is usually a yellow-red margin visible between the pink normal nail and the white separated area. In the 'oil spot' or 'salmon patch' variety, the separation between nail plate and nail bed may start in the middle of the nail; this is sometimes surrounded by a yellow margin,

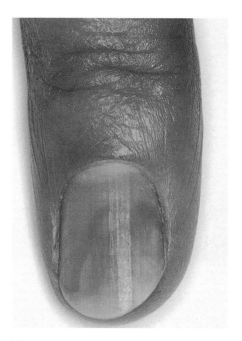

Figure 4.1
Onycholysis.

especially in psoriasis. The accumulation of large amounts of serum-like exudate containing glycoprotein, in and under the affected nails, explains the colour change in this condition. Glycoprotein is also commonly found in

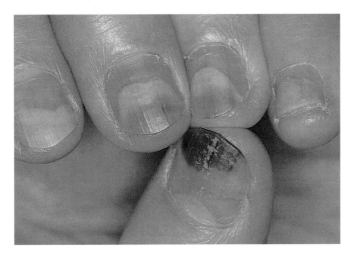

Figure 4.2
Onycholysis with *Pseudomonas aeruginosa* discoloration.

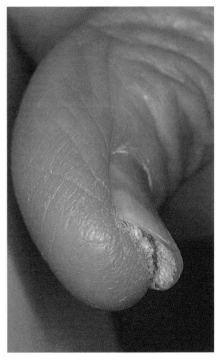

Figure 4.3
Onycholysis – showing the separation of the nail plate and nail bed.

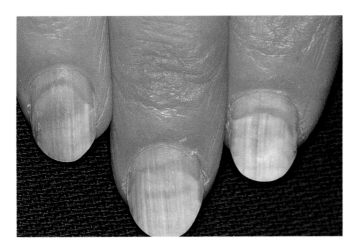

Figure 4.4
Onycholysis due to psoriasis.

inflammatory and eczematous diseases affecting the nail bed. Oil patches have been reported in systemic lupus erythematosus; they may be extensive in lectitis purulenta et granulomatosa.

Onycholysis is usually symptomless. The extent of onycholysis increases progressively and can be estimated by measuring the distance separating the distal edge of the lunula from the proximal limit detachment. Transillumination of the terminal phalanx gives a good view of the affected area. The onset may be sudden in trauma (often of occupational origin) and in photo-onycholysis (Figure 4.5) where there may be a triad of photosensitization, onycholysis and dyschromia. Four distinct types of onycholysis (often preceded by onychodynia) were noted after both antibiotics

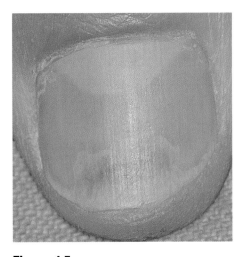

Figure 4.5
Photo-onycholysis.

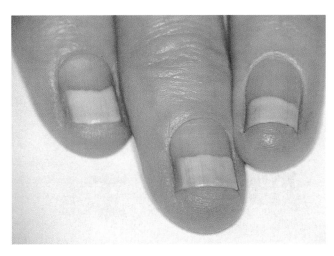

Figure 4.6
Self-induced onycholysis.

and psoralens were administered; one common sign was prevalent in the first three types: the lateral margins of the nails were unaffected.

- Type I: several fingers are involved; the separating part of the nail plate is half-moon-shaped and concave distally with a pigmentation of variable intensity, and shows a well-demarcated proximal border.
- Type II: one finger only is affected; a well-defined circular notch is present, which opens distally and has a brownish hue proximally.
- Type III: in the central part of the pink nail bed on several fingers, there is initially a round yellow staining that turns reddish after 5–10 days.
- Type IV: bullae under the nails have been reported in photo-onycholysis due to tetracycline hydrochloride and in four types of cutaneous porphyria – porphyria cutanea tarda, erythropoietic porphyria, erythropoietic protoporphyria and variegate porphyria – as well as in pseudo-porphyria.

Sudden onset of oncholysis may also be due to contact with chemical irritants such as hydrofluoric acid or hair remover containing thioglycolate. In finger nails, irregularly sculptured onycholysis is a self-induced nail abnormality due to excessive manicure with a sharp instrument (Figure 4.6). Sometimes the proximal lytic border is straight or gently curved.

Onycholysis of the toe demonstrates some differences from the condition on the fingers: the major distinctions are due to:

- The lack of occupational causes.
- The reduced use of cosmetics on the toes.
- The protection afforded by footwear (photo-onycholysis is rare).

The two main causes of onycholysis of the toe nail, especially the great toe nail, are onychomycosis and traumatic onycholysis. Onycholysis of the great toe nail is often seen when the second toe overrides it. Other causes

> **Finger nail onycholysis as an isolated sign on a few nails in adult women is often perpetuated by overzealous manicuring**

Table 4.1 Some causes of onycholysis

Idiopathic
   Leuko-onycholysis paradentotica (Schuppli syndrome)
   Of women (cosmetic use)

Systemic
   Circulatory (e.g. lupus erythematosus)
   Yellow nail syndrome
   Endocrine (e.g. hypothyroidism, thyrotoxicosis)
   Pregnancy
   Syphilis
   Iron deficiency anaemia
   Carcinoma of the lung
   Pellagra

Congenital and/or hereditary
   Partial hereditary onycholysis
   Pachyonychia congenita

Cutaneous diseases
   Psoriasis, Reiter's disease, vesicular or bullous disease, lichen planus, alopecia areata,
      multicentric reticulohistiocytosis
   Atopic dermatitis, contact dermatitis (accidental or occupational), mycosis fungoides, actinic
      reticuloid
   Hyperhidrosis – tumours of the nail bed

Drugs
   Bleomycin, docetaxel, doxorubicin, fluorouracil, retinoids, captopril, paclitaxel, mitozantrone
   Drug-induced photo-onycholysis: trypaflavin, chlorpromazine, chloramphenicol, cephaloridine,
      icodextrin, clorazepate dipotassium, allopurinol, cloxacillin (exceptional), tetracyclines:
      especially demethylchlortetracycline and doxycycline, also minocycline, fluoroquinolones,
      photochemotherapy with psoralens (sunlight or PUVA), thiazide diuretics, flumequine,
      quinine, oral contraceptives, indomethacin, captopril

Local causes
   Trauma (accidental, occupational, self-inflicted (Figure 4.6) or mixed) as with clawing,
      pinching or stabbing
   Foreign bodies
   Infection
      Fungal
      Bacterial
      Viral (e.g. warts, herpes simplex, herpes zoster)
   Chemical irritants (accidental or occupational)
      Prolonged immersion in (hot) water with alkalis and/or detergents, sodium hypochlorite, etc.
      Paint removers
      Sugar solution
      Gasoline and similar solvents
      Cosmetics (formaldehyde, false nails, depilatory products, nail polish removers); nickel
         derived from metal pellets in nail varnish
   Physical
      Thermal injury (accidental or occupational)
      Microwaves

are onychogryphosis and, in children, congenital malalignment of the hallux nails. In fungal oncholysis, primary *Candida* infection is almost exclusively confined to the finger nails. In distal subungual onychomycosis of the toe nails, the horny thickening raises the free edge with secondary disruption of the attachment of the nail plate to the nail bed. The nail bed epithelium is irreversibly transformed into epidermis, thus prohibiting reattachment of the nail.

Primary candidal oncholysis is almost exclusively confined to the finger nails. In distal subungual onychomycosis of the toe nails, the horny thickening raises the free edge of the nail with disruption of the normal nail plate–nail bed attachment: this gives rise to secondary oncholysis. Some authors have questioned whether great toe nail onychomycosis is ever truly primary. Its presence should always lead to a search for abnormalities of the foot such as hyperkeratosis of the metatarsal heads, thickening of the ball of the foot or pressure on the great toe by an overriding second toe.

Table 4.1 lists many potential causes of oncholysis. The most common types presenting to dermatologists are due to psoriasis, onychomycosis and the cosmetic 'sculptured' varieties of adult women.

ONYCHOMADESIS AND SHEDDING

Nails may be shed by the progression of any severe type of oncholysis causing the nail plate to separate more proximally (Figures 4.7–4.12). Onychomadesis is the spontaneous separation of the nail plate from the matrix area; this is associated with some arrest of nail growth (see the section on transverse lines, Chapter 3). At first a split appears under the proximal portion of the nail, followed by the disappearance of the juxtamatricial portion of the surface of the nail. A surface defect is thus

formed, which does not usually involve the deeper layers. It is due to a 'limited' lesion of the proximal part of the matrix. In latent onychomadesis the nail plate shows a transverse split because of transient, complete inhibition of nail growth for a minimum of 1–2 weeks. It may be characterized by a Beau's line which has reached its maximum dimensions, although the nail continues growing for some time because there is no disruption in its attachment to the underlying tissues. Growth ceases when it is shed after losing this connection. In some severe, general acute diseases, such as Lyell's syndrome, the proximal edge of all the nail plates may be elevated. Growth proceeds because of the continued movement of the nail bed to which the nails remain attached (Figures 4.7–4.9).

The terms 'onychoptosis defluvium' or 'alopecia unguium' are sometimes used to describe traumatic nail loss. Onychomadesis usually results from serious generalized diseases, bullous dermatoses, drug reactions, intensive X-ray therapy, acute paronychia or severe psychological stress; or it may be idiopathic. Nail shedding may be an inherited disorder (as a dominant trait); the shedding may be periodic, and rarely associated with the dental condition amelogenesis imperfecta. Longitudinal fissures, recurrent onychomadesis and onychogryphosis can be associated with mild degrees of keratosis punctata. Minor traumatic episodes (as in 'sportsman's toe') may cause onychomadesis of the toe nails (Figure 4.12).

Retronychia has been described in patients with acute onychomadesis involving individuals with a 3–6 months' history of inflammation of the affected digits. After ineffective conservative treatment avulsion revealed three generations of nail joined distally but separated proximally, with the upper and oldest generation embedded into the overlying proximal nail fold. Failure of longitudinal growth, combined with the wedge-like effect of the new nail beneath, directed the overlying nail upwards

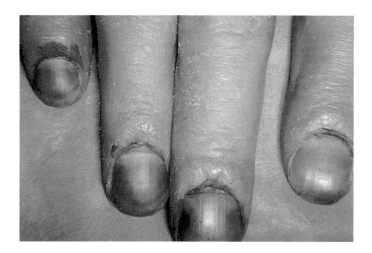

Figure 4.7
Lyell's syndrome – early proximal
changes.

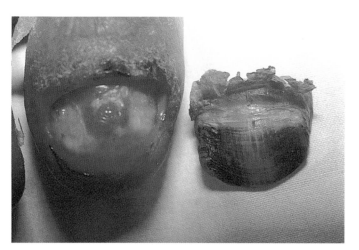

Figure 4.8
Lyell's syndrome – nail shedding.
(Courtesy of S. Goettmann.)

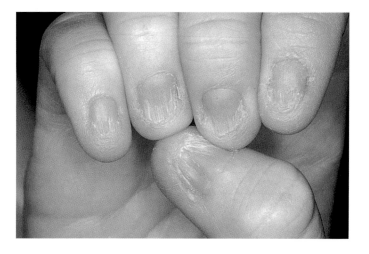

Figure 4.9
Lyell's syndrome – nails shed and
permanent scarring. (Courtesy of S.
Goettmann.)

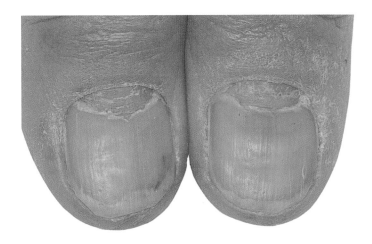

Figure 4.10
Onychomadesis due to psoriasis.

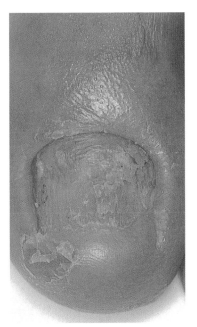

Figure 4.11
Nail shedding due to pustular psoriasis.

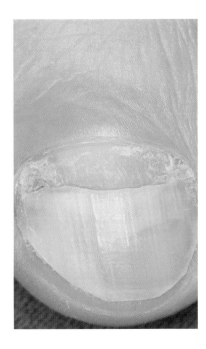

Figure 4.12
Post-traumatic onychomadesis.

into the proximal nail fold. This non-recurrent condition resolves through loss of the nail.

Total nail loss with scarring may be due to permanent damage of the matrix following trauma, or the late stages of acquired onychatrophy following lichen planus, bullous diseases or chronic peripheral vascular insufficiency. In texts on congenital anomalies this defect is sometimes referred to as aplastic anonychia, which does not always produce scarring. Temporary, total nail loss may also result from severe progressive onycholysis.

Table 4.2 lists many of the recognized causes of nail shedding.

Table 4.2 Causes and associations of nail shedding

Local inflammation, e.g. acute paronychia
    (Figures 4.7–4.12)
Kawasaki's syndrome
Fever or systemic upsets
Syphilis
Bullous dermatoses, e.g. pemphigus
Stevens–Johnson syndrome
Toxic epidermal necrolysis (Lyell's syndrome)
    (Figures 4.7–4.9)
Drugs
    Cytotoxics
    Antibiotics
    Retinoids
Keratosis punctata
Local trauma
X-irradiation
Acrodermatitis enteropathica
Hypoparathyroidism with amelogenesis
    imperfecta
Yellow nail syndrome

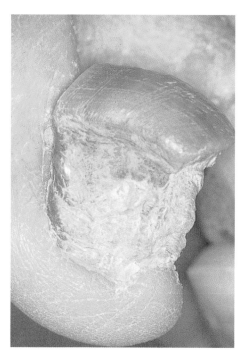

Figure 4.13
Cryptogenic hyperkeratosis.

HYPERTROPHIC NAIL AND SUBUNGUAL HYPERKERATOSIS

Ideally, the term 'hypertrophy of the nail plate' should be restricted to conditions causing nail enlargement and thickening by their effects on the nail matrix (excluding nail bed and hypony-chium). The term 'subungual hyperkeratosis' should relate to those entities leading to thick-ening beneath the preformed nail plate: that is, thickening of the nail bed or hyponychium (Figure 4.13). In practice, this differentiation is difficult to define and mixed cases are commonly seen, for example in psoriasis (Figures 4.14, 4.15).

The normal thickness of finger nails is approximately 0.5 mm; this is consistently increased in manual workers and in many disease states such as congenital ichthyoses, Darier's disease, psoriasis and repeated trauma. The latter particularly relates to toe nails where microtrauma and footwear are constantly affecting the nails.

Onychogryphosis (Figures 4.16–4.18), a condition mainly seen in the great toe nails of elderly and infirm individuals, is probably due to trauma, footwear pressure, neglect and sometimes associated poor peripheral circula-tion and fungal infection; these and less common causes are listed in Table 4.3.

If the nail bed is left continuously exposed by nail removal or disease for more than a few months irregular hyperkeratosis and failure of nail plate adhesion may ensue

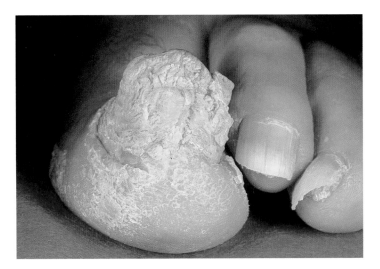

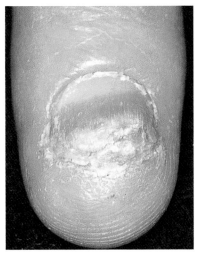

Figure 4.14
Subungual hyperkeratosis due to psoriasis.

Figure 4.15
Distal subungual hyperkeratosis in psoriasis; note proximal inflammatory brown margin.

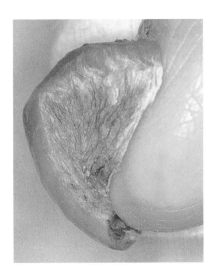

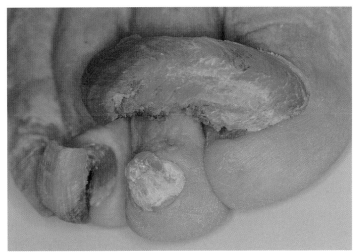

Figure 4.16
Oyster-like onychogryphosis.

Figure 4.17
Onychogryphosis – ram's horn deformity.

Epithelial hyperplasia of the subungual tissues results from repeated trauma and exudative skin diseases and may occur with any chronic inflammatory condition involving this area. It is especially common in psoriasis, pityriasis rubra pilaris and chronic eczema and may also be due to fungi (Figures 4.19–4.25). Histological investigation reveals periodic acid–Schiff reagent (PAS)

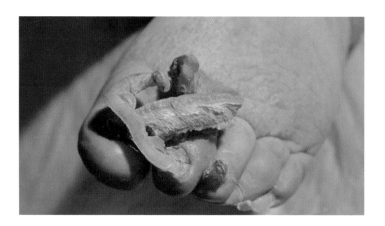

Figure 4.18
Severe onychogryphosis.

Table 4.3 Causes and associations of onychogryphosis

Dermatological
    Ichthyosis
    Psoriasis
    Onychomycosis
    Syphilis, pemphigus, variola

Local causes
    Isolated injury to the nail apparatus
    Repeated minor trauma caused by
        footwear
    Foot faults such as hallux valgus

Regional causes
    Associated varicose veins
    Thrombophlebitis (even in the upper limb)
    Aneurysms
    Elephantiasis
    Disease involving the peripheral nervous
        system

General causes
    Old age
    Vagrancy and senile dementia
    Disease involving the central nervous
        system
    Hyperuricaemia

Idiopathic forms
    Acquired or hereditary

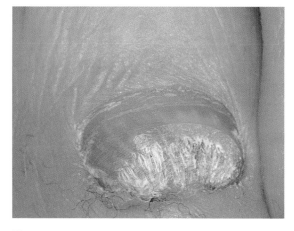

Figure 4.19
Subungual hyperkeratosis due to *Trichophyton rubrum* infection.

positive, homogeneous, rounded or oval, amorphous masses surrounded by normal squamous cells which are usually separated from each other by empty spaces caused by the fixation process. These clumps, which coalesce and enlarge, have been described in psoriasis of the nail, onychomycosis, eczema and alopecia areata, and also in some hyperkeratotic processes such as subungual warts and pincer nails. The horny excrescences of the nail bed are not very obvious, but the ridged structure may become apparent if the nail plate is cut and shortened.

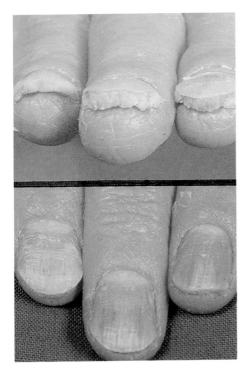

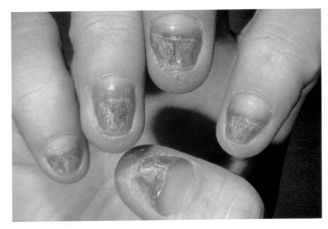

Figure 4.21
Hypertrophic, hard nail in pachyonychia congenita.

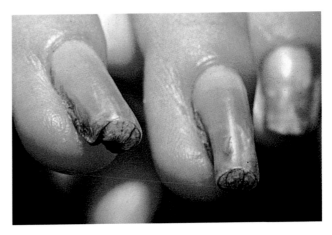

Figure 4.20
Subungual hyperkeratosis due to pityriasis rubra pilaris. (Courtesy of R. Caputo, Milan.)

Figure 4.23
Pachyonychia congenita – marked distal subungual thickening. (Courtesy of C. Beylot, Bordeaux.)

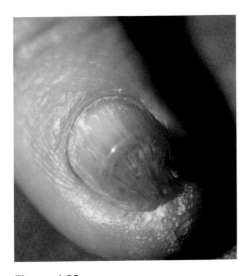

Figure 4.22
Pachyonychia congenita.

In keratosis cristarum the keratinizing process is limited to the peripheral area of the nail bed. It starts at the distal portion but may progress somewhat proximally. *Scopulariopsis brevicaulis* onychomycosis may present with similar changes.

Table 4.4 lists the causes of thick nails often associated with onycholysis; Table 4.5 lists the causes of thick nails and/or subungual hyperkeratosis.

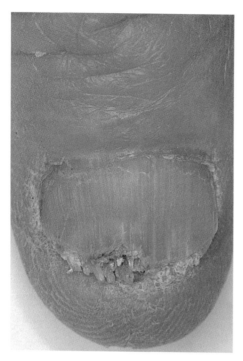

Figure 4.24
Subungual hyperkeratosis due to lichen planus.

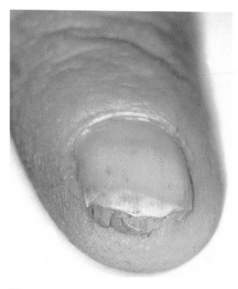

Figure 4.25
Darier's disease – distal, irregular, subungual
thickening.

Table 4.4 Causes of thick nails (often associated with onycholysis)

Psoriasis/Reiter's syndrome (Figures 4.14, 4.15)
Onychomycosis (Figure 4.19)
Pityriasis rubra pilaris (Figure 4.20)
Pachyonychia congenita (Figures 4.21–4.23)
Contact eczema
  Mineral oils
  Cement
  Hair styling products
Acrokeratosis paraneoplastica (Bazex's
  syndrome)
Lichen planus
Yellow nail syndrome

Table 4.5 Causes of thick nails and/or subungual hyperkeratosis

Frequent
  Onychomycosis (Figure 4.19)
  Psoriasis (Figures 4.14–4.15)
  Contact eczema
    Mineral oils
    Cement
    Hair styling products
  Repeated microtrauma
  Single major trauma
  Subungual clavus

Less frequent
  Bowen's disease
  Lichen planus (Figure 4.24)
  Norwegian scabies
  Pachyonychia congenita (Figures 4.21–4.23)
  Pityriasis rubra pilaris (Figure 4.20)
  Acrokeratosis paraneoplastica (Bazex's
    syndrome)
  Reiter's syndrome
  Darier's disease (Figure 4.25)
  Erythroderma
  Ichthyosis
  Sezary's syndrome
  Onychopapilloma of the nail bed

Rare
  Alopecia areata
  Radiodermatitis
  Arsenic keratosis

SPLINTER HAEMORRHAGES AND HAEMATOMAS

Splinter haemorrhages

The subungual epidermal ridges extend from the lunula distally to the hyponychium and fit 'tongue and groove' fashion between similarly arranged dermal ridges. The disruption of the fine capillaries along these longitudinal dermal ridges results in splinter haemorrhages (Figures 4.26–4.29).

Macroscopically, splinter haemorrhages appear as tiny linear structures, usually no more than 2–3 mm long, arranged in the long

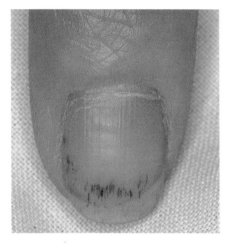

Figure 4.26
Splinter haemorrhages.

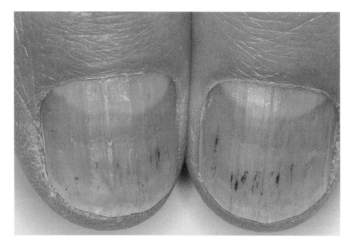

Figure 4.27
Psoriatic distal subungual splinter haemorrhages.

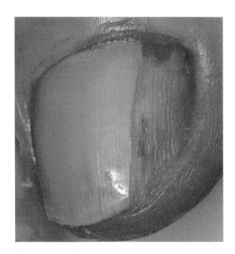

Figure 4.28
Sites of splinter haemorrhages in the nail bed.

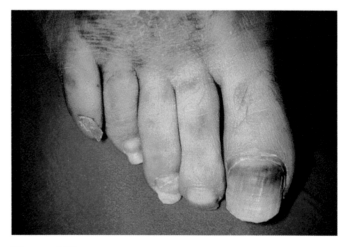

Figure 4.29
Subungual haemorrhage in vitamin C deficiency (scurvy). (Courtesy J. J. Grob, Marseilles.)

Table 4.6 Causes of splinter haemorrhages

Amyloidosis
Antiphospholipid syndrome
Arterial emboli
Arthritis (notably rheumatoid arthritis and
    rheumatic fever)
Behçet's syndrome
Blood dyscrasias (severe anaemia, high-
    altitude purpura)
Buerger's disease
Cirrhosis
Collagen vascular disease
Cryoglobulinaemia (with purpura)
Darier's disease
Drug reactions (especially tetracyclines)
Eczema
Haemochromatosis
Haemodialysis and peritoneal dialysis
Heart disease (notably uncomplicated mitral
    stenosis and subacute bacterial
    endocarditis)
High-altitude living
Histiocytosis X
Hypertension
Hypoparathyroidism
Idiopathic (probably traumatic) – up to 20%
    of normal population
Indwelling brachial artery cannula
Malignant neoplasia
Occupational hazards
Onychomatricoma
Onychomycosis
Palmoplantar keratoderma
Peptic ulcer
Pityriasis rubra pilaris
Psoriasis
Pterygium
Pulmonary disease
Radial artery puncture
Raynaud's disease
Renal disease
Sarcoidosis
Scurvy
Septicaemia
Severe illness
Thyrotoxicosis
Minor and repeated trauma
Trichinosis
Vasculitis

axis of the nail. The majority originate within the distal third of the nail from the 'spirally wound' capillary which produces the pink line normally seen through the nail about 4 mm proximal to the tip of the finger. When splinter haemorrhages originate from the proximal portion of the nail accompanied by a longitudinal xanthonychia, the diagnosis of onychomatricoma should be considered. Splinter haemorrhages rarely involve the whole nail bed. When first formed they are plum-coloured but darken to brown or black within 1–2 days; subsequently they move superficially and distally with the growth of the nail, and at this stage they can be scraped from the undersurface of the nail plate. The nature of splinter haemorrhages is not clearly known. They may result from emboli in the terminal vessels of the nail bed; the emboli may be septic, or due to trauma of various types; they are more common in the first three fingers of both hands, and develop at the line of separation of the nail plate from the nail bed. Familial capillary fragility may cause splinter haemorrhages in otherwise healthy individuals. Occasional haemorrhages are of no clinical significance and are probably traumatic. There is a statistically greater incidence of splinter haemorrhages in men than in women, and in black compared with white individuals. In healthy women they are usually confined to a single digit. Histochemical studies of nail parings confirm that the linear discoloration is derived from blood. The blood pigments give a negative Prussian blue and Pearls' reaction.

Many conditions may be associated with splinter haemorrhages (Table 4.6). In all cases it is probable that, whatever the pathogenesis, the nail bed capillaries are more susceptible to minor trauma leading to linear haemorrhages.

Haematomas

Small haemorrhages originating in the nail bed remain subungual as growth progresses distally. The deeper layers of the nail are stained by small pockets of dried blood entrapped in the nail plate. Those produced by trauma to the more proximal part of the matrix will appear in the upper layers of the plate. Sometimes patches of leukonychia overlie the haematoma. Moderate trauma to the nail area, or blood dyscrasias, affecting extensive numbers of dermal ridges, determine whether the haemorrhages are punctate or result in large ecchymoses. Acute subungual haematomas are usually obvious, occurring shortly after trauma involving finger or toe nails. The blood which accumulates beneath the nail plate produces pain which may be severe. Haematomas are also discussed in Chapter 9.

> **Traumatic subungual toe nail haemor-rhage may be entirely painless**

The technique used for drainage depends on the size and site of the haematoma. Treatment is required to prevent both unnecessary delay in the regrowth of the nail plate and secondary dystrophy which might result from pressure on the matrix due to accumulated blood under the nail. In acute haematoma of the proximal nail area, drainage of the haematoma with a fine-point scalpel blade or by drilling a hole through the plate will give prompt relief from pain. Hot paper-clip cautery is a useful alternative to trephining the plate. This allows blood to be evacuated; the nail is then pressed against the bed by a moderately tight bandage, helping the nail plate to readhere. If this procedure is not immediately practicable, the pain can be relieved by elevating the limb and maintaining the position for approximately 30 minutes.

Occasionally subungual haematoma persists under the nail and does not migrate. A reddish-blue colour, irregular shape, and the absence of colour in the nail plate help to differentiate non-migrating subungual haematomas from naevi and other causes of nail pigmentation. It is advisable to remove the part overlying the subungual haematoma and identify and remove the dried blood in order to establish the diagnosis and to exclude more significant disease such as malignant melanoma.

In total haematoma, often observed when there is injury to the nail bed, the possibility of an underlying fracture must be considered: radiographic investigation is therefore neces-sary. The nail is removed, the haematoma evacuated and the wound repaired, if neces-sary with precise suturing of the nail bed using 6-0 polyglycolic acid or polydioxane sutures. The plate is then cleaned, shortened, narrowed and held in place by suturing to the lateral nail folds. The stitches are removed after 10 days, and usually the nail remains firmly attached.

The differential diagnosis of subungual blood from melanin may be difficult. The haemor-rhage is between the nail plate and the matrix and nail bed epithelium, and is entrapped by the regrowing nail; the blood is not therefore degraded to haemosiderin by macrophages, and is not positive to Prussian blue staining. It can, however, easily be demonstrated: a small amount of the pigmented material is scraped from the nail plate undersurface and, collected in a test tube, a few drops of water are added and a reagent strip is dipped into it to test for the presense of haemoglobin. A positive test indicates the presence of blood.

Subungual bleeding may be due to many systemic conditions; Table 4.7 lists the most common morphological types.

DORSAL AND VENTRAL PTERYGIUM

Dorsal pterygium consists of a gradual exten-sion of the proximal nail fold over the nail plate (Figures 4.30–4.32). The nail plate becomes fissured because of the fusion of the proximal

Table 4.7 Splinter haemorrhages and subungual haematoma in some systemic conditions

	Haematoma	Splinters
Arterial lines/puncture	–	+
Bacterial endocarditis	–	+
Blood dyscrasia	+	+
Cirrhosis	–	+
Collagen vascular disease	+	+
Cryoglobulinaemia	–	+
Drugs	–	+
Dialysis	–	+
Emboli	+	+
Histiocytosis X (Langerhans cell histiocytosis)	–	+
Scurvy	+	+
Sepsis	–	+
Thyroid	–	+
Vasculitis	–	+

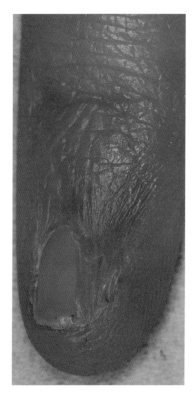

Figure 4.30
Post-traumatic pterygium (lateral longitudinal biopsy).

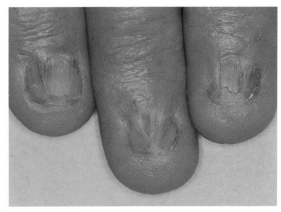

Figure 4.31
Pterygium at different stages in lichen planus.

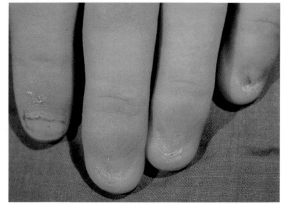

Figure 4.32
Pterygium – terminal stage in lichen planus.

nail fold epidermis to the nail bed; its split portions progressively decrease in size as the pterygium widens. This often results in two small nail remnants if the pterygium process is

central. Complete involvement of the matrix and nail bed in the pathological process leads to total loss of the nail plate, with permanent atrophy and scarring in the nail area (see

Pterygium is a wing-shaped scar and is always irreversible

onychatrophy, page 35). Dorsal pterygium is particularly seen in scarring lichen planus; less often in peripheral ischaemia, severe bullous dermatoses, and radiotherapy on the hands of radiologists; it may follow injury; rarely, congenital forms occur.

Ventral pterygium, or pterygium inversum unguis (Figure 4.33), is a distal extension of the hyponychial tissue which anchors to the undersurface of the nail, thereby eliminating the distal groove. Scarring in the vicinity of the distal groove, causing it to be obliterated, may produce secondary pterygium inversum unguis. Ventral pterygium may be seen in scleroderma associated with Raynaud's phenomenon, disseminated lupus erythematosus, and causalgia of the median nerve. The condition may be idiopathic, congenital, and familial or acquired. A congenital, aberrant, painful hyponychium has been described associated with oblique, deep fractures of the nails. In one case an unusual acquired association of pterygium inversum unguis and lenticular atrophy of the palmar creases was recorded.

Pain in the finger tip from minor trauma and haemorrhages may appear when the distal, subungual area is repeatedly pushed back or the nail cut short. Toe nails are only rarely involved. Subungual pterygium (non-inflammatory) is analogous to the claw of lower primates. In patients suffering from dorsal pterygium (excluding the traumatic or congenital types) the main characteristic is dilatation in the nail fold

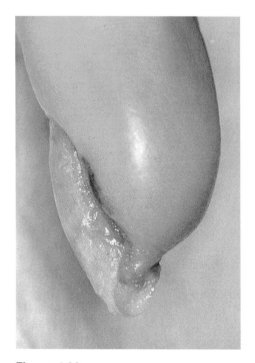

Figure 4.33
Ventral pterygium in acrosclerosis.

Table 4.8 Causes of pterygium

Dorsal
 Congenital
 Bullous dermatoses (e.g. cicatricial
  pemphigoid, Stevens–Johnson syndrome)
 Burns
 Dyskeratosis congenita
 Graft-versus-host disease
 Lichen planus (most common cause)
 Onychotillomania
 Radiodermatitis
 Raynaud's disease and peripheral vascular
  disease

Ventral
 Congenital
 Familial
 Formaldehyde nail hardeners
 Idiopathic
 Peripheral neuropathy
 Raynaud's disease and systemic sclerosis
 Trauma

capillary loops and the formation of a slender microvascular shunt system in the more dilated loops. These changes are visible by capillaroscopy. Table 4.8 lists the well-recognized causes of pterygium. Lichen planus is the most common specific cause of dorsal pterygium. Ventral pterygium is most frequently seen in association with Raynaud's disease and systemic sclerosis.

FURTHER READING

Achten G, Wanet-Rouard J (1970) Pachyonychia, *Br J Dermatol* **83**: 56–62.

Baran R (1986) Les onycholyses, *Ann Dermatol Vénéréol* **113**: 159–170.

Baran R, Badillet G (1982) Primary onycholysis of the big toenails. A review of 113 cases, *Br J Dermatol* **106**: 526–534.

Baran R, Juhlin L (2002) Photoonycholysis, *Photodermatol Photoimmunol Photomed* **18**: 202–207.

Caputo R, Cappio F, Rigon C *et al* (1993) Pterygium inversum unguis. Report of 19 cases and review of the literature, *Arch Dermatol* **129**: 1307–1309.

DePaoli RT, Marks VJ (1987) Crusted (Norwegian) scabies: treatment of nail involvement, *J Am Acad Dermatol* **17**: 136–138.

Kechijian P (1985) Onycholysis of the fingernails: evaluation and management, *J Am Acad Dermatol* **12**: 552–560.

Ray L (1963) Onycholysis, *Arch Dermatol Syphil* **88**: 181.

Runne V, Orfanos CE (1981) The human nail, *Curr Prob Dermatol* **9**: 102–149.

Sonnex TS, Dawber RPR, Zachary CB *et al* (1986) The nails in type I pityriasis rubra pilaris: a comparison with Sezary syndrome and psoriasis, *J Am Acad Dermatol* **15**: 956–960.

5 Periungual tissue disorders

Robert Baran

Paronychia · Ragged cuticles and hangnail · Painful dorsolateral fissures of the finger tip · Tumours and swellings · Pustules · Miscellaneous dermatoses · Further reading

PARONYCHIA

The proximal nail fold, with its distal cuticle attached to the nail and the ventral eponychium, is normally well adapted to prevent infections and external inflammatory agents entering the proximal matrix area; the same is true of the lateral nail walls and folds. It is therefore probable that no paronychia is truly primary, there always being some physical or chemical damage preceding the infection or inflammation; this is less true in relation to superficial infections on the dorsum of the proximal nail fold, such as 'bulla repens' (a bullous form of impetigo).

Acute paronychia

Minor trauma is a frequent cause of acute paronychia and surgical treatment may be necessary. Infection may follow a break in the skin (for example, if a hangnail is torn), a splinter under

> **Acute paronychia needs urgent systemic antibiotic treatment to prevent permanent nail dystrophy**

the distal edge of the nail, a prick from a thorn in a lateral groove, or sometimes from subungual infection secondary to haematoma (Figures 5.1, 5.2).

The infection begins in the lateral paronychial areas with local redness, swelling and pain. At this stage medical treatment is indicated: wet compresses (for example with Burrow's aluminium acetate solution) and appropriate systemic antibiotic therapy are given. Because the continuation of antibiotics may mask a developing pathological process that can damage the nail apparatus, if acute paronychia does not show clear signs of response within 2 days then surgical treatment should be instituted under proximal block local anaesthesia. The purulent reaction may take several days to localize and during this time throbbing pain is always a major symptom. The collection of pus may easily be seen through the nail or at the paronychial fold. Sometimes a bead of pus may be present in the periungual groove. In the absence of visible pus, the gathering gives rise to tension and the lesion should be incised at the site of maximum pain, not necessarily at the site of maximum swelling. In practice, Bunell's technique is usually successful: the base of the nail (the proximal third) is removed by cutting across with pointed scissors. A non-adherent gauze wick is laid under the proximal nail fold. If the

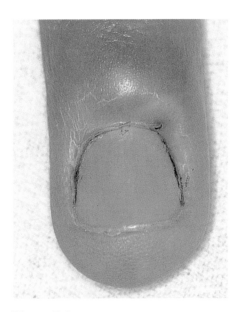

Figure 5.1
Acute bacterial paronychia.

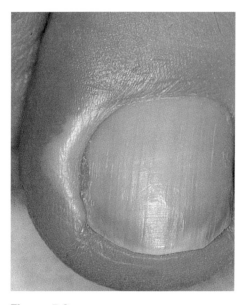

Figure 5.2
Acute bacterial paronychia – pus
tracking within the lateral nail fold.

paronychial infection remains restricted to one side, removal of the ipsilateral part of the nail is sufficient.

Bacterial culture and sensitivity studies are mandatory. The bacteria most commonly found in acute paronychia are staphylococci and, less commonly, β-haemolytic streptococci and Gram-negative enteric bacteria. Should surgical intervention be delayed, the pus will track around the base of the nail under the proximal nail fold and inflame the matrix; it may then be responsible for transient or permanent dystrophy of the nail plate. It is essential to note that the nail matrix in early childhood is particularly fragile and can be destroyed within 48 hours by acute bacterial infection. The pus may also separate the nail from its loose, underlying proximal attachment. The firmer attachment of the nail at the distal border of the lunula may temporarily limit the spread of the pus. In cases with extension of the infection under the distal nail bed, the whole of the

nail base should be removed with nail removed distally to expose fully the involved nail bed.

Distal subungual pyogenic infection may or may not be secondary to the periungual varieties. Treatment is by excision of a U-shaped piece of the distal nail plate in the region loosened by the pus and debridement of the affected nail bed. Extension of the infection may involve the finger pulp or the matrix. Sometimes the evacuation of a perionychial phlyctenular abscess uncovers a narrow sinus; this may be part of a 'collar-stud' abscess which communicates with a deeper, necrotic zone; it must be exposed and excised. If acute paronychia accompanies ingrowing nail, the treatment must be supplemented by removing all offending portions of the nail plate. After surgery, the dressing is kept moist with saline or an antiseptic soak. This should be changed daily after bathing in antiseptic soap until the purulent discharge stops – preferably with full splinting and immobilization of finger, hand and forearm.

In general, acute paronychia involves only one nail. In chronic or subacute paronychia, which may mimic acute paronychia, several finger nails may be infected. The differential diagnosis includes:

- paronychial inflammation of the finger nails accompanying chronic eczema
- herpes simplex (Figure 5.37)
- psoriasis and Reiter's disease, which may also involve the proximal nail fold
- acute ischaemia where the finger is cold.

Chronic paronychia

Chronic paronychia is an inflammatory disorder of the proximal nail fold, typically affecting hands that are continually exposed to a wet environment and repeated minor trauma causing cuticle damage. When the cuticle is torn or lost, the epidermal barrier of the proximal nail fold is impaired and the nail fold is then exposed to a large number of environmental hazards. Irritants and allergens may easily penetrate the proximal nail fold and produce contact dermatitis that is responsible for the chronic inflammation. A variety of immediate hypersensitivity (type I) reaction to food ingredients may be seen. Sometimes irritant reaction may precede it.

The condition is prevalent in people in contact with water, soap, detergents and other chemicals (Figure 5.3); it is particularly associated with housework. There is also a high incidence among chefs, bartenders, confectioners and fishmongers. The index and middle finger of the left hand are most often affected, these being the digits most subject to minor trauma such as rubbing during hand-washing

> **Chronic paronychia is not a primary infection**

> **Chronic paronychia of the hands is typically initiated by frequent immersion of hands in water**

of clothes. Clinically, the proximal and lateral nail folds show erythema and swelling. The cuticle is lost and the ventral portion of the proximal nail fold becomes separated from the nail plate. This newly formed space has an important additional role in maintaining and aggravating chronic paronychia – it becomes a receptacle for micro-organisms and environmental particles that potentiate the chronic inflammation. With time the nail fold retracts and becomes thickened and rounded.

The course of chronic paronychia is interspersed with self-limiting episodes of painful acute inflammation. The acute exacerbations of chronic paronychia may be due to secondary

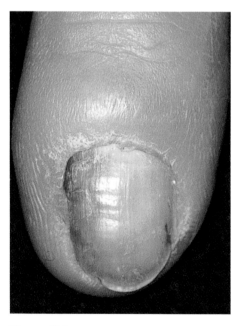

Figure 5.3
Chronic paronychia due to constant wetting.

candidal and bacterial infections, with small abscesses resulting at the depth of the space between the proximal nail fold and the nail plate. These microbial abscesses drain spontaneously and this explains why such bacterial exacerbations subside without treatment in a few days.

Acute exacerbations of chronic paronychia are not only due to microbial colonization, but can also be caused by irritants or allergens that penetrate deep to the proximal nail fold. In occupational paronychia, foreign material such as wax, hair, foodstuffs and debris may collect in the proximal nail fold. This may cause retraction of the nail fold and persistence of the process. In the early stages the nail plate is unaffected, but one or both lateral edges may develop irregularities and yellow, brown or blackish discoloration; this may extend over a large portion of the nail, and occasionally the whole nail may become involved. It is believed to follow discoloration caused by dihydroxyacetone produced by the organisms in the nail fold. In contrast, *Pseudomonas* infection often produces a greenish discoloration. The lateral discoloured edges of the nail plate become cross-ridged when the disease mainly affects the lateral nail fold. On the surface, which often becomes rough and friable, numerous irregular transverse ridges or waves appear as a result of repeated acute exacerbations. Eventually the size of the nail is considerably reduced, an effect exaggerated by the swelling of the surrounding soft tissues. The pathology of chronic paronychia reveals spongiotic dermatitis of the ventral portion of the proximal nail fold.

There is some disagreement as to the importance of yeasts in chronic *Candida* paronychia; this organism may be commensal or pathogenic. *Candida* hypersensitivity is a similar reaction to that observed in some patients with recurrent vaginitis.

The various factors that damage the area allow *Staphylococcus aureus* and *Candida* species to attack the keratin and cause the detachment of the cuticle from the nail plate. In children the most common predisposing factor to chronic candidal paronychia is the habit of thumb or finger sucking. This is potentially more harmful than occupational immersion, as saliva is more irritating than water. Paronychia may also develop in people with eczema or psoriasis involving the nail folds. Although infrequent, chronic paronychia of the toe nails may develop in association with diabetes mellitus or peripheral vascular disease, both of which should be excluded unless ingrowing nail is present.

Differential diagnosis

Chronic paronychia can be associated with nail infections caused by various species of *Scytalidium*. Brown discoloration starting at the lateral edges of the nail and spreading centrally into the nail is seen in some cases. Rarely this is caused by separate *Candida* infection which is not directly related to the original *Scytalidium* infection. In white people, *Fusarium oxysporum* may produce chronic paronychia in finger or toe nails.

Syphilitic paronychia is due to a chancre on the perionychial area; it is usually painful. Pemphigus may produce considerable bolstering of the nail fold and closely resembles chronic paronychia with accompanying onychomycosis. Parakeratosis pustulosa (Hjorth–Sabouraud syndrome) may also mimic fungal paronychia. Psoriatic lesions, Reiter's syndrome and eczema sometimes involve the proximal nail fold. Secondary bacterial or yeast infections may develop in the area.

Treatment

If chronic paronychia becomes recalcitrant and unresponsive to medical procedures, most often after penetration of foreign bodies such as hair, bristle or wood splinters, then surgical removal of the proximal nail fold and proximal lateral nail folds together with the proximal nail plate may be required; after this procedure complete healing normally takes approximately 8 weeks.

Table 5.1 shows the principal causes of paronychia (Figures 5.1–5.11). Acute paronychia is most commonly seen in nail biters, while the most frequently seen type of chronic paronychia is that occurring on the hands of domestic and office cleaners and bar staff (wet work) (see Figure 5.3).

Table 5.1 Causes of paronychia

Infective
  Acute
    Viral
    Bacterial (Figures 5.1, 5.2)
    Fungal
    Parasitic
  Chronic
    Mycotic (Figure 5.3)
    Mycobacterial
    Syphilitic

Drugs
  Retinoids (Figures 5.4, 5.5)

Cosmetic
  Trauma
  Epoxy resin dermatitis

Occupational (Figure 5.3)

Dermatoses
  Acrodermatitis enteropathica (Figure 5.6)
  Contact dermatitis
  Darier's disease
  Dyskeratosis congenita
  Eczema
  Hallopeau's acrodermatitis
  Ingrowing toe nail
  Lichen planus

Pachyonychia congenita
Parakeratosis pustulosa
Pemphigus
Psoriasis–Reiter's syndrome (Figure 5.7, 5.8)
Radiodermatitis
Yellow nail syndrome

Systemic disease
  Antiretroviral drugs
  Cytotoxic drugs
  Collagen vascular diseases (Figure 5.9)
  Encephalitis
  Frostbite
  Histiocytosis X
  Ischaemia (acute)
  Leukaemia
  Metastases
  Neuropathy
  Paraneoplastic acrokeratosis
  Sarcoidosis (Figure 5.10)
  Stevens–Johnson syndrome
  Toxic epidermal necrolysis
  Vasculitis
  Zinc deficiency (Figure 5.11)

Miscellaneous
  Finger-sucking in children
  Foreign body granuloma

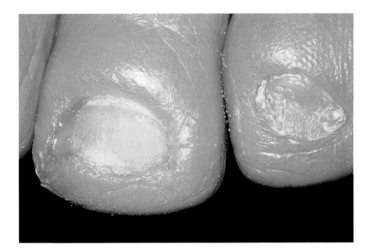

Figure 5.4
Chronic paronychia due to oral
etretinate therapy.

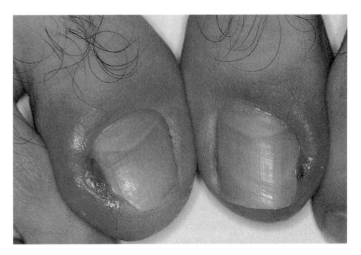

Figure 5.5
Chronic paronychia with
granulation tissue due to oral
isotretinoin therapy.

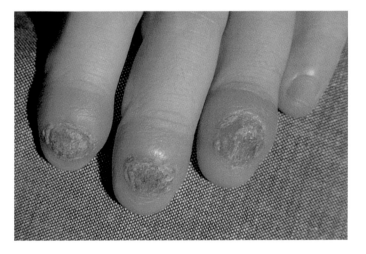

Figure 5.6
Chronic paronychia in
acrodermatitis enteropathica.
(Courtesy of Professor Bourlond.)

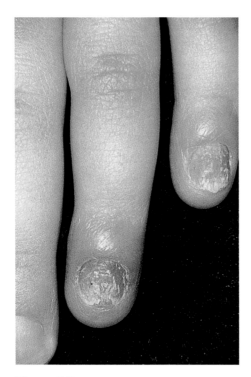

Figure 5.7
Chronic paronychia in psoriasis.

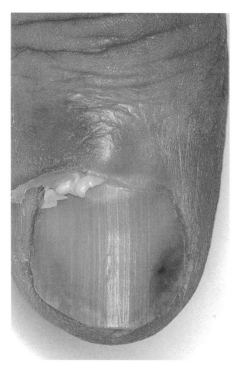

Figure 5.8
Chronic paronychia in psoriasis.
Squeezing the nail fold produces a
cheesy material (Sabouraud's medium
negative).

Figure 5.9
Paronychial inflammation due to
systemic lupus erythematosus.

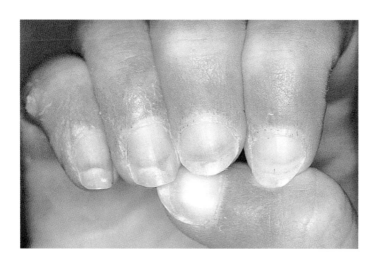

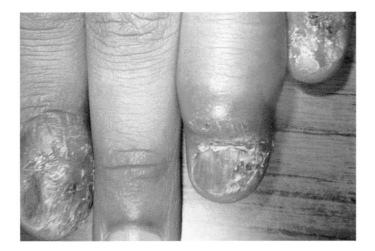

Figure 5.10
Chronic granulomatous paronychia due to sarcoidosis. (Courtesy of J. Hewitt.)

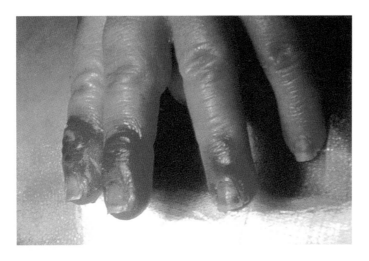

Figure 5.11
Paronychia due to zinc deficiency.

RAGGED CUTICLES AND HANGNAIL

Thickened, hyperkeratotic, irregular (ragged) cuticles (Figure 5.12) are most commonly seen in dermatomyositis (Figure 5.13). Perionychial tissues are constantly subjected to trauma. In nail biters and 'pickers' the cuticles and nail folds may show considerable damage, erosions, haemorrhage and crusting. The ulnar side of the nail fold and cuticle is most vulnerable and there may be small triangular tags of skin (hangnail, Figure 5.14) and separated spicules of nail, still attached proximally. Thickened cuticle composed of several layers (onion-like) can be an unusual manifestation of factitious damage.

Hangnails may also result from occupational injuries, due to the hydration and dehydration caused by frequent wetting. However, usually hangnail has no obvious cause, though it may be self-induced.

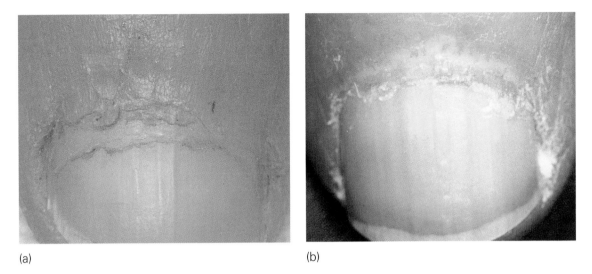

(a)   (b)

Figure 5.12
Ragged cuticles: (a) unknown cause; (b) scleroderma.

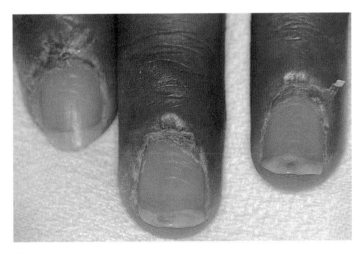

Figure 5.13
Dermatomyositis with ragged cuticles.

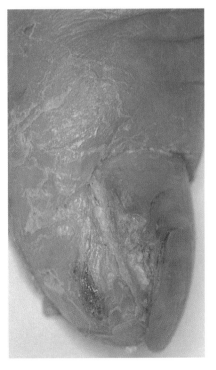

Figure 5.14
Hangnail deformity of the lateral nail.

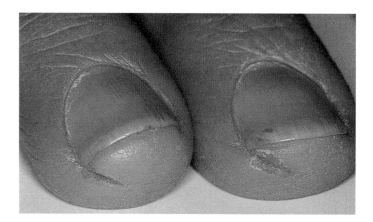

Figure 5.15
Dorsolateral fissures – usually very painful.

PAINFUL DORSOLATERAL FISSURES OF THE FINGER TIP

In individuals with dry skin, particularly in winter, painful dorsolateral fissures may be seen located distal to the lateral nail groove (Figure 5.15). This has been observed mainly in psoriasis and atopic dermatitis.

TUMOURS AND SWELLINGS

Table 5.2 lists some of the nore common lesions in relation to their site in the nail apparatus. Benign and malignant lesions are detailed in Table 5.3. The nail apparatus develops *in utero* from primitive skin and it is therefore not surprising that many of the swellings and tumours that affect the rest of the skin can occur within it. Table 5.4 lists the vast array of such conditions which have been described in and around the nail apparatus; only the distinctive lesions that are peculiar to the nail apparatus and those that have different morphology in this site are described in detail.

Periungual and subungual warts

Common warts are caused by human papillomaviruses of different biological types (Figures 5.16–5.18). They are benign, weakly infective,

Table 5.2 Tumours of the nail unit (by site)

At the nail fold/plate junction
Acquired periungual fibrokeratoma
Periungual fibroma (tuberous sclerosis)

Within the nail fold
Myxoid pseudocysts
Tendon sheath giant cell tumour

On the nail folds and nail walls
Verruca vulgaris
Recurring digital fibrous tumour of
childhood

Within the nail bed with or without nail plate destruction
Subungual exostosis
Osteochondroma
Enchondroma
Subungual corn (heloma)
Pyogenic granuloma
Glomus tumour
Recurring digital fibrous tumour of
childhood
Bowen's disease and squamous cell
carcinoma
Melanoma
Metastases

Table 5.3 Differential diagnosis of subungual malignant melanoma

Malignant lesions	Benign lesions
Pigmented	**Longitudinal melanonychia**
Haemangioendothelioma	Melanocytic hyperplasia
Kaposi's sarcoma	Junctional naevus
Metastatic melanoma	Adrenal insufficiency
	Adrenalectomy for Cushing's disease
	Angiokeratoma
	Chromogenic bacteria (*Proteus*)
	Drugs: antimalarials, cytotoxics, arsenic, silver, thallium, phenothiazines and PUVA
	Haematoma, trauma
	Irradiation
	Laugier–Hunziker–Baran syndrome
	Onychomycosis nigricans
Amelanotic	
Basal cell carcinoma	Epidermal cyst
Bowen's disease	Exostosis
Squamous cell carcinoma	Foreign body granuloma
Metastasis	Onychomatricoma Keratoacanthoma
	Pyogenic granuloma
	Ingrowing nail

PUVA, psoralens with long-wave ultraviolet irradiation.

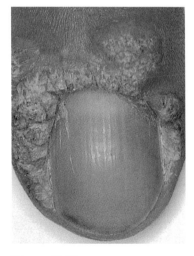

Figure 5.16
Periungual viral warts.

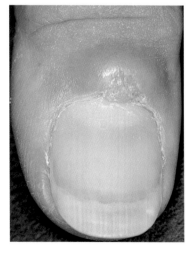

Figure 5.17
Smaller proximal nail fold due to viral wart.

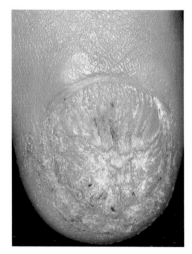

Figure 5.18
Subungual viral wart with nail plate destruction.

Table 5.4 Tumours and swellings affecting the nail apparatus (those in bold type are described in the text)

Warts	**Glomus tumour**
Verrucous epidermal naevus	Pyogenic granuloma
Subungual papilloma	Naevus flammeus and angioma
Subungual onychopapilloma	Angiokeratoma circumscriptum
Verrucous lesions in incontinentia pigmenti	Aneurysmal bone cyst (arteriovenous fistula)
Subungual corn	**Osteochondroma Subungual exostosis**
Epidermoid cyst	Enchondroma
Onychomatricoma	Maffucci's syndrome
Fibromatous lesions	Osteoid osteoma
Keloids	Hereditary multiple exostosis (diaphyseal aclasis)
Dermatofibroma	**Myxoid pseudocyst**
Koenen's tumour	Myxoma
Acquired periungual fibrokeratoma	**Bowen's disease**
Subungual filamentous tumour	**Squamous cell carcinoma**
Benign juvenile digital fibromatosis	**Keratoacanthoma**
Leiomyoma	Basal cell carcinoma
Giant cell tumour	Sarcoma
Xanthoma	Kaposi's sarcoma
Lipoma	Lymphoma
Neurogenic tumours	Metastases
Multicentric reticulohistocytosis	**Melanotic/melanocytic lesions**
Actinic keratosis	Benign melanocytic hyperplasia
Arsenical keratosis	Lentigo simplex and naevocytic naevus
	Atypical melanocytic hyperplasia
	Peutz–Jeghers–Touraine syndrome
	Malignant melanoma
	Laugier–Hunziker–Baran syndrome

fibro-epithelial tumours with a rough keratotic surface. Usually periungual warts are asymptomatic, although fissuring may cause pain. Subungual warts initially affect the hyponychium, growing slowly toward the nail bed and finally elevating the nail plate. Bone erosion from verruca vulgaris occasionally occurs – although some of these cases may have been keratocanthomas, since the latter, epidermoid carcinoma and verruca vulgaris are sometimes indistinguishable by clinical signs alone.

Subungual warts are painful and may mimic glomus tumour. The nail plate is not often affected, but surface ridging may occur and, more rarely, dislocation of the nail. Biting, picking and tearing of the nail and nail walls are common habits in people with periungual warts. This type of trauma is responsible for the spread of warts and their resistance to treatment.

Tuberculosis cutis verrucosa (butcher's nodule) may rarely pose differential diagnostic problems, but it is unusual in the periungual location, affecting a lateral fold of the toe nails with long-standing warty lesions with unusual wart morphology. Bowen's disease must be considered, as should the subcutaneous vegetations of systemic amyloidosis.

Treatment of periungual warts is often frustrating. Treatments with X-rays and radium have become obsolete. Saturated monochloroacetic acid has been suggested, but is painful; it is applied sparingly, allowed to dry and then covered with 40% salicylic acid plaster cut to the size of the wart and held in place with adhesive tape for 2–3 days. After 1–2 weeks many of the warts can be removed and the procedure repeated. Subungual warts are treated similarly, after cutting away the overlying part of the nail plate. Recalcitrant warts may respond to weekly applications of diphencyprone solutions ranging from 0.2% to 2%, according to the patient's ability to produce a good inflammatory reaction. Some authorities recommend the use of cantharidin (0.07%); this is applied to the lesions and covered by a plastic tape for 24 h. The resultant blister should be retreated at 2-week intervals, three to four times if necessary. Bleomycin has also been recommended for recalcitrant warts; it is given intralesionally 1 μg per ml at 2-week intervals. Some patients find this more painful than correctly used cryosurgery.

Surgical treatment should be avoided if possible. Cryosurgery with carbon dioxide snow or liquid nitrogen is often used but may cause blistering, with the blister roof containing the epidermal wart component if the treatment succeeds. However, when treating the proximal nail fold freezing must not be prolonged since the matrix can easily be damaged; this may result in circumscribed leukonychia or even nail dystrophy, although scarring is rare with cryosurgery. Particular side-effects of cryosurgery include pain, depigmentation and secondary bacterial infection (rare), Beau's lines, onychomadesis, nail loss or inordinate oedema, the latter often worse in the very young and very old, and transient neuropathy or anaesthesia. Many of the side-effects are avoidable if the freezing times are carefully controlled and if prophylactic analgesic and subsequent anti-inflammatory treatment is given: soluble aspirin 600 mg three times daily for 5 days and topical steroid application twice daily. Destruction by curettage and electrodesiccation may produce considerable scarring. Infrared coagulation and argon and carbon dioxide laser treatments have been used with some success. If the most aggressive measures fail, or compliance is poor, formalin may be applied daily with a wooden toothpick. If the lesions become inflamed, fissured or tender, because of the therapy or secondary infection, treatment is interrupted and a topical antiseptic preparation used for several days. Many people have tricks for attempting to cure warts, such as 'wrapping', followed 2 weeks later by the careful application of liquefied phenol, then a drop of nitric acid to the lesion. The fuming and spluttering that occurs looks efficacious, and the wart turns brown.

Since the incubation period of human warts may be up to several months, consistent follow-up, even after seemingly successful therapy, is necessary to allow for early treatment of newly growing warts.

Onychomatricoma

Four main clinical signs characterize onychomatricoma, a recently identified tumour specific to the nail apparatus, with finger nails being much more often affected than toe nails:

- A yellow longitudinal band of variable width, leaving a single or double portion of normal pink nail on either side.
- Splinter haemorrhages involving the proximal nail region.
- A tendency toward transverse overcurvature of the nail.
- Nail avulsion exposes a villous tumour emerging from the matrix while the nail plate appears as a thickened funnel, storing the filamentous digitations fitting into the holes of its proximal extremity.

Interestingly, some clinical presentations may be confusing: for example, a longitudinal melanonychia may hide the yellow hue. A swelling at the junction of the proximal nail fold and the lateral nail fold may produce the appearance of cutaneous horn, sometimes completely separated from the nail plate. Associated onychomycosis may be misleading also. Magnetic resonance images are typical and allow confirmation of the clinical diagnosis (see p. 98).

Histological examination shows multiple 'glove finger' digitations lined with matrix epithelium oriented around antero-oblique connective tissue axes, and perforation of the nail plate by multiple cavities which (generally at the distal edge of the lunula) lose their epithelial digitations and become filled with serous fluid. The connective tissue stroma of the digitations extends deeply into the dermis and is not demarcated from healthy tissue.

Fibromas

Many different types of fibroma may occur in and around the nail (Figure 5.19). They may be true entities or merely variants of one process.

Keloids

Hypertrophic scars and keloids result from injuries to the nail fold or nail bed and may significantly distort the nail apparatus.

Dermatofibroma

Nail apparatus dermatofibromas are rare and may resemble cutaneous horns, fibrokeratomas or supernumerary digits; the latter, however, usually arise on the ulnar aspect of the fifth metacarpophalangeal joint. The histological changes include areas of thick, hypocellular, hyalinized collagen bundles, randomly orientated; there is an ill-defined nodule situated mainly in the reticular dermis; elastic fibres are often scarce or absent.

Koenen's tumour

Koenen's periungual fibromas develop in 50% of cases of tuberous sclerosis (epiloia or Bourneville–Pringle disease). They usually appear at about 12–14 years of age and increase progressively in size and number with

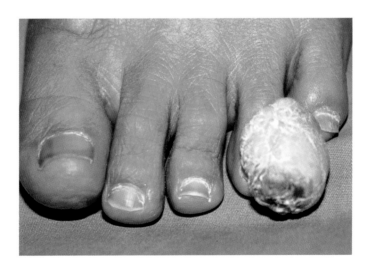

Figure 5.19
Periungual fibroma. (Courtesy of Akiro Kamumochi, Japan.)

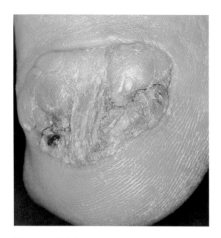

Figure 5.20
Koenen's tumour associated with nail plate destruction.

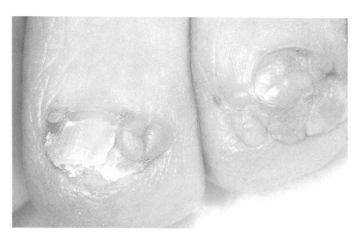

Figure 5.21
Multiple Koenen's tumours.

age. Individual tumours are small, round, flesh-coloured and asymptomatic, with a smooth surface (Figures 5.20, 5.21). The tip may be slightly hyperkeratotic, resembling fibrokeratoma. The tumors grow out from the nail fold, eventually overgrowing the nail bed and destroying the nail plate. Depending on their site of origin, they may cause longitudinal depressions in the nail plate. Excessively large tumours are often painful, requiring excision. Histological changes consist of dense angiofibrotic tissue, sometimes with neuroglial tissue at the centre, and hyperkeratosis at the tip.

Koenen's tumours are cured by simple excision. Usually no suture is necessary. Tumours growing out from under the proximal nail fold are removed after reflecting the proximal nail fold back by making lateral incisions down each margin in the axis of the lateral nail grooves. Subungual fibromas are removed after avulsion of the corresponding part of the nail plate.

Acquired periungual fibrokeratoma

Acquired periungual fibrokeratomas are probably identical to acquired digital fibrokeratomas and Steel's 'garlic clove' fibroma. They are acquired, benign, spontaneously developing, asymptomatic nodules with a hyperkeratotic tip and a narrow base (Figures 5.22, 5.23). They most commonly occur in the periungual area or on other parts of the fingers. A case was described in which the lesion was located beneath the nail, visible under the free margin of the great toe nail. Most periungual fibrokeratomas emerge from the most proximal part of the nail sulcus growing on the nail and causing a sharp longitudinal depression. Trauma is thought to be a major factor initiating acquired periungual fibrokeratoma.

Microscopically, acquired periungual fibrokeratomas resemble hyperkeratotic 'dermal hernias'. The core consists of mature eosinophilic collagen fibres oriented along the main vertical axis of the tumour. The fibroblastic cells are increased in number. Most fibromas are highly vascular. The epidermis is thick and acanthotic. There is a marked orthokeratotic horny layer, which may be parakeratotic and contains serum or blood at the tip of the tumour. Elastic fibres are normal. Acid mucopolysaccharide levels are not increased.

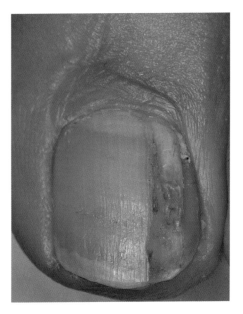

Figure 5.22
Acquired fibrokeratoma.

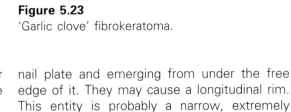

Figure 5.23
'Garlic clove' fibrokeratoma.

Surgical treatment is the same as for Koenen's tumours and depends on the size and location of the lesion.

The differential diagnosis of acquired periungual fibroma includes:

- keloid
- Koenen's tumour
- recurring digital fibrous tumours of childhood
- dermatofibrosarcoma
- fibrosarcoma
- acrochordon
- cutaneous horn
- eccrine poroma
- pyogenic granuloma
- verruca vulgaris
- exostosis.

Subungual filamentous tumour

Subungual filamentous tumours are thread-like, horny, subungual lesions growing with the nail plate and emerging from under the free edge of it. They may cause a longitudinal rim. This entity is probably a narrow, extremely hyperkeratotic fibrokeratoma; it can be pared down painlessly when the nail is cut.

Recurring digital fibrous tumours of childhood (benign juvenile digital fibromatosis)

Recurring digital fibrous tumours are round, smooth, firm tumours with a reddish or livid red colour. They are located on the dorsal and axial surfaces of the fingers and toes, characteristically sparing the thumbs and great toes (Figure 5.24). They may present at birth or develop during infancy, although a single case of presentation in adulthood has been described. There is no sex predominance. Fingers are more often affected than toes. On reaching the nail unit the tumours may elevate the nail plate, leading to dystrophy but not to

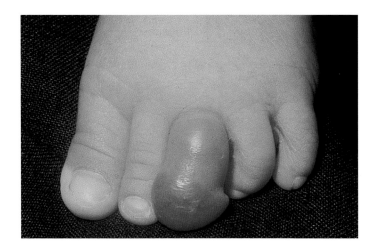

Figure 5.24
Benign juvenile digital fibromatosis
(Courtesy of C. Moss, UK.)

destruction. Often the tumour is multicentric, occurring on several digits. Although an infectious origin is probable, no virus has been isolated and viral particles have not been demonstrated by electron microscopy. Up to 60% recur after excision. Spontaneous regression was noted in 5 out of 61 cases; regression may be hastened by cryosurgery. Radical surgical ablation of the area involved may rarely be necessary, including the nail unit, leading to permanent loss of the nail. Firm plantar nodules may be associated with these tumours.

Histological examination shows a diffuse, proliferative, cellular process in the dermis with increased numbers of apparently normal fibroblasts with uniform, spindle-shaped nuclei. Mitoses are absent or rare. Elastic tissue is decreased. In about 2% of the fibroblasts, paranuclear inclusion bodies, 3–10 μm in diameter, can be seen in adequately fixed specimens with the use of stains such as iron haematoxylin, methyl green–pyronin and phosphotungstic acid–haematoxylin. Electron microscopy shows that the inclusions consist of fibrillar masses without a limiting membrane. On the basis of this evidence, it has been suggested that the condition should be termed 'elastodysplasia'.

Distal digital keratoacanthoma

Subungual and periungual keratoacanthomas may occur as solitary or multiple tumours. They are rare, benign, rapidly growing, seemingly aggressive tumours usually situated beneath the distal portion of the nail bed. The lesion starts as a small, painful keratotic nodule visible beneath the free edge, growing rapidly to a 1 cm lesion within 4–8 weeks. Its typical gross appearance, as a dome-shaped nodule with a central plug of horny material filling the crater, is more obvious on an adequate histological specimen. Less frequently the tumour grows out from under the proximal nail fold, which becomes swollen and inflamed. In contrast to keratoacanthomas elsewhere, in distal digital tumors, spontaneous regression is rare.

The tumour soon erodes the bone, but reconstitution of the defect can be achieved.

Glomus tumour

The glomus tumour was first described about 200 years ago as a painful, subcutaneous 'tubercle'. Several cases were described as 'malignant angiosarcomas' or 'colloid sarco-mas'. Seventy-five per cent of glomus tumours occur in the hand, especially in the finger tips and particularly the subungual area. Between 1% and 2% of all hand tumours are glomus tumours. The age at the time of diagnosis ranges from 30 years to 50 years. Men are less frequently affected than women.

The tumour is characterized by intense, often pulsating pain that may be spontaneous or provoked by the slightest trauma. Even changes in temperature, especially from warm to cold, may trigger pain radiating up to the shoulder. Sometimes the pain is worse at night: it may disappear when a tourniquet is applied.

The tumour is seen through the nail plate as a small, bluish to reddish-blue spot several millimetres in diameter, rarely exceeding 1 cm (Figure 5.25). Sometimes it causes a slight rise in surface temperature which can be detected by thermography. Minor nail deformities are caused by 50% of the tumours – ridging or a nail plate 'gutter' being the most common. A similar proportion cause a depression on the dorsal aspect of the distal phalangeal bone, or even a cyst visible on X-ray. Probing, which elicits pain, and transillumination may help to localize the tumour if it is not clearly visible through the nail. If the tumour cannot be local-ized clinically or by X-ray, arteriography should be performed; this will reveal a star-shaped telangiectatic zone. In selected cases, magnetic resonance imaging (MRI) has been shown to help in the diagnosis of a glomus tumour of the finger tip, revealing even very small lesions.

Many patients give a history of trauma. The most common misdiagnoses are neuroma, causalgia, gout and arthritis. Histological exami-nation shows a highly differentiated, organoid tumour. It consists of an afferent arteriole, vascular channels lined with endothelium and surrounded by irregularly arranged cuboidal cells with round, dark nuclei and pale cytoplasm. Primary collecting veins drain into the cutaneous veins. Myelinated and non-myelinated nerves are found and may account for the pain. The tumour is surrounded by a fibrous capsule. Since all the elements of the normal glomus are present, the glomus tumour may be considered as a hamartoma rather than a true tumour.

Treatment is by surgical excision. Small tumours may be removed by punching a 6 mm hole in the nail plate, incising the nail bed and enucleating the lesion. The small nail disc is put back in its original position as a physiolog-ical dressing. Larger tumours may be treated after removal of the proximal half of the nail plate; those in lateral positions are removed by an L-shaped incision parallel to and 4–6 mm on the volar side of the lateral nail fold. The nail bed is carefully dissected from the bone until the tumour is reached and removed. This is usually curative, although the pain may take

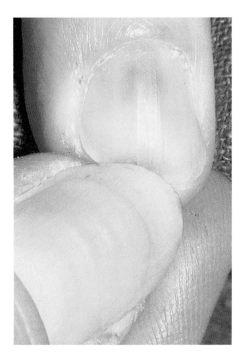

Figure 5.25
Glomus tumour.

several weeks to disappear. Recurrences occur in 10–20% of cases and may represent incomplete excision or adjacent tumours overlooked at the initial operation, or genuine new growth. More extensive surgery than is usual might achieve more first-time cures.

Subungual exostosis

Subungual exostoses are not true tumours but rather outgrowths of normal bone or calcified cartilaginous remains (Figure 5.26). Whether or not subungual osteochondroma is a different entity is not clear. Subungual exostoses are painful bony growths which elevate the nail. They are particularly frequent in young people and are mostly located in the great toe, although less commonly subungual exostoses also occur on the fingers. They start as small elevations of the dorsal aspect of the distal phalanx and eventually emerge from under the nail edge or destroy the nail plate. If the nail is

> **Distorted nail shape may be due to a bone tumour**

shed, the surface becomes eroded and secondarily infected, sometimes mimicking ingrown toe nail. Walking may be painful.

Trauma appears to be a major causative factor, although some authors claim that a history of trauma only occurs in a minority. The triad of pain (the leading symptom), nail deformation and radiographic features is usually diagnostic. The exostosis is a trabeculated osseous growth with an expanded distal portion covered with radiolucent fibrocartilage.

Osteochondroma, commonly presenting with the same symptoms, has a male predominance. There is often a history of trauma. Its growth rate is slow. Radiographic examination shows a well-defined, sessile, bony growth with a hyaline cartilage cap which must be differentiated from primary subungual calcification (particularly in

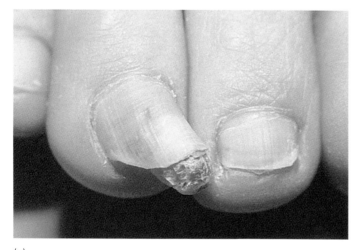
(a)

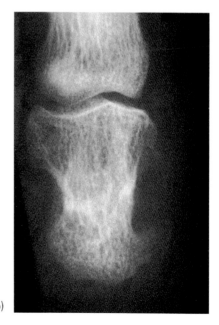
(b)

Figure 5.26
(a) Exostosis; (b) X-ray of exostosis.

older women) and secondary subungual calcification due to trauma and psoriasis.

Treatment is by excision of the excess bone under full aseptic conditions. The nail plate is partially removed and a longitudinal incision made in the nail bed. The osseous growth with its cartilaginous cap is carefully dissected, using fine skin hooks to avoid damage to the fragile nail bed. The tumour is removed with a fine chisel, whenever possible through an L-shaped or 'fish mouth' incision, in order to avoid avulsion of the nail plate.

Myxoid pseudocysts of the digits

The many synonyms for mixed pseudocyst of the digits reflect the controversial nature of this lesion:

- dorsal finger cyst
- synovial cyst
- recurring myxomatous cyst
- cutaneous myxoid cyst
- dorsal distal interphalangeal joint ganglion
- digital mucinous pseudocyst
- focal myxomatous degeneration
- mucoid cyst.

Whereas some authors regard it as a synovial cyst, most now believe it to be a periarticular degenerative lesion.

Myxoid cysts occur more often in women. They are typically found in the proximal nail fold of the fingers and rarely on toes (Figures 5.27–5.29). Usually asymptomatic, these lesions vary from soft to firm, cystic to fluctuant, and may be dimpled, dome-shaped or smooth-surfaced. Transillumination confirms their cystic nature. They are always located to one side of the midline and rarely exceed

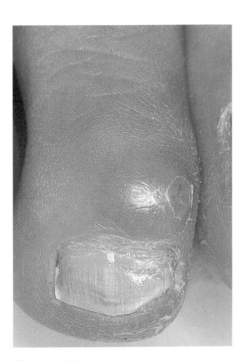

Figure 5.27
Large periungual myxoid pseudocyst.

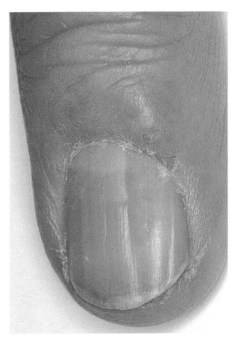

Figure 5.28
Nail plate gutter due to myxoid pseudocyst.

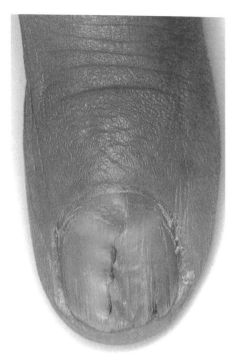

Figure 5.29
Subungual myxoid pseudocyst with nail plate disruption.

10–15 mm in diameter. The skin over the lesion is thinned and may be verrucous or even ulcerated. Rarely, a paronychial fistula may develop under the proximal nail fold, less commonly under the nail plate. Longitudinal grooving of the nail results from pressure on the matrix. Occasionally a series of irregular transverse grooves are seen, suggesting alternating intermittent decompression and refilling of the cyst. Degenerative, 'wear and tear' osteoarthritis, frequently with Heberden's nodes, is present in most cases.

Histopathological investigation reveals the pseudocystic character. Cavities without synovial lining are located in an ill-defined fibrous capsule. The structure is essentially myxomatous with interspersed fibroblasts. Areas of myxomatous degeneration may merge to form a multilocular pseudocyst. In

> **Myxoid pseudocysts rarely occur without 'wear and tear' osteoarthritis**

the cavities, a jelly-like substance is found which stains positively for hyaluronic acid. In some cases a mesothelial-like lining is found in the stalk connecting the pseudocyst with the distal interphalangeal joint. It has been suggested that the lesion arises from the joint capsule or tendon sheath synovia, as do ganglia in other areas.

A multitude of treatments have been recommended, including repeated incision and drainage, simple excision, multiple needlings and expression of contents, X-irradiation (5 Gy, 50 kV, Al 1mm, three times at weekly intervals), electrocautery, chemical cautery with nitric acid, trichloroacetic acid or phenol, massages or injection of proteolytic substances, hyaluronidase, steroids (fluorandrenolone tape, or injections) and sclerosing solutions, cryosurgery, radical excision and even amputation.

The intralesional injection of corticosteroid crystal suspension has been recommended. The cyst is first drained from a proximal point to avoid leakage of the steroid suspension when the patient's hand is lowered. Careful dissection and excision of the lesion gives the highest cure rate. A tiny drop of methylene blue solution, diluted with a local anaesthetic solution and mixed with fresh hydrogen peroxide, is injected into the distal interphalangeal joint at the volar joint crease. The joint will accept only 0.1–0.2 ml of dye. This clearly identifies the pedicle connecting the joint to the cyst, if one is present, and also the cyst itself. This procedure sometimes reveals occult satellite cysts.

Alternatively, the methylene blue may be injected into the cyst to define the tract back to its site of origin. The incision line is drawn on the finger, including a portion of the skin directly over the cyst and continuing proximally in a gentle curve to end dorsally over the joint. The lesion is meticulously dissected from the surrounding soft tissue and the pedicle traced to its origins adjacent to the joint capsule and resected. Dumb-bell extension of cysts to each side of the extensor tendon is easily dissected by hyperextending the joint. Osteophytic spurs adjacent to the joint must be removed with a fine chisel or bone rongeur. Liquid nitrogen cryosurgery has been used with an 86% cure rate. The field treated included the cyst and the adjacent proximal area to the transverse skin creases overlying the terminal joint. Two freeze/thaw cycles were carried out, each freeze time being 30 s after the ice field had formed, the intervening thaw time being at least 4 min; if this method is adopted then longer freeze times must be avoided or permanent matrix damage may occur. If the cyst is first pricked and emptied of its gelatinous contents, then equally good cure rates can be obtained with a single 20 s freeze after initial ice formation. For distal posterior nail fold lesions, excision of the proximal nail fold and associated cyst has been recommended.

Sclerosing agents may also be useful: after puncture and expression of cyst contents 0.20–0.30 ml of a 1% solution of sodium tetradecyl sulphate is injected; a second or a third injection may be required at monthly intervals.

Bowen's disease (epidermoid carcinoma)

Bowen's disease is a term for intra-epithelial squamous carcinoma (Figures 5.30–5.32). It is not as rare as might be inferred from the medical literature.

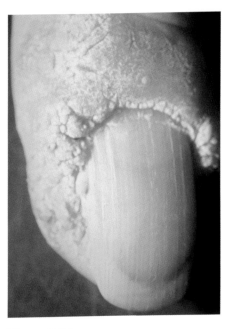

Figure 5.30
Epidermoid carcinoma – verrucous periungual involvement.

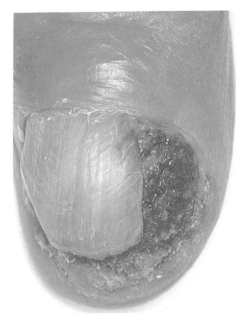

Figure 5.31
Epidermoid carcinoma – subungual involvement.

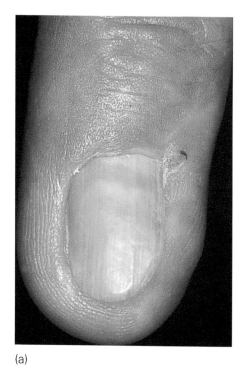

(a)

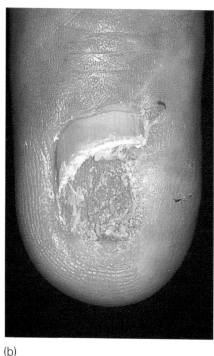

(b)

Figure 5.32
(a) Epidermal carcinoma; (b) epidermal carcinoma, with nail plate trimmed back to show extension of invasion. (Courtesy of G. Cannata, Italy.)

The clinical picture of Bowen's disease of the nail unit is variable. It may show a periungual erythematous, squamous or eroded plaque. In the lateral nail wall and groove, it usually presents as a recalcitrant hyperkeratotic or papillomatous, slowly enlarging lesion. Distal involvement of the proximal nail fold results in the formation of a characteristic whitish band. The fingers are far more frequently affected than the toes: typically the thumbs, less often the index and middle fingers. The median age at presentation is approximately 60 years, men predominating. Bowen's disease evolves and expands only slowly. Biopsies taken from the most indurated and warty area often reveal invasive squamous

cell carcinoma in contrast to the flat plaque. Many authorities therefore no longer differentiate Bowen's disease from squamous cell carcinoma, preferring the term 'epidermoid carcinoma' for all cases.

Surgical removal of the affected area and a small margin of healthy tissue is the treatment of choice. With some authorities, we prefer the Mohs fresh tissue removal method. Despite the fact that cryosurgery is highly effective in treating Bowen's disease at other skin sites, it is only rarely effective for nail apparatus types.

> **Intra-epithelial squamous carcinoma is not rare, the whole tumour usually having local invasion at some point**

Squamous cell carcinoma

Squamous cell carcinoma of the nail unit (also known as epidermoid carcinoma) is a low-grade malignancy. Many cases have been reported, with a male predominance.

> **Squamous cell carcinoma of the nail apparatus has a good prognosis compared with other sites**

Trauma, chronic infection and chronic radiation exposure are possible aetiological factors; human papillomavirus (HPV) has been incriminated in some cases. Two reported cases had associated congenital ectodermal dysplasia. Most lesions occur on the fingers, particularly the thumbs and index fingers (Figure 5.31). The presenting symptoms include pain, swelling, inflammation, elevation of the nail, ulceration, a tumour 'mass', ingrowing of the nail, 'pyogenic granuloma' and bleeding. Bone involvement is a rare, very late sign. The duration of symptoms before diagnosis is greater than 12 months in over half the cases. Only in one published case (with ectodermal dysplasia) has the condition led to death, from rapid generalized metastases.

Subungual squamous cell carcinoma is slow-growing and may be mistaken for chronic infection. This frequent misdiagnosis unduly prolongs the period between the onset of the disease, diagnosis and therapy. Often it is not possible to determine whether the tumour was present initially or developed later, secondary to trauma, warts or infection. As mentioned above, invasive squamous cell carcinoma may develop from Bowen's disease. The possibility of a link with HPV strains 16, 34 and 35 sheds new light on the aetiology of this type of cancer and suggests a logical cause for multiple digital Bowen's disease.

Subungual melanotic lesions

The term 'longitudinal melanonychia' (LM) describes the presence of single or multiple

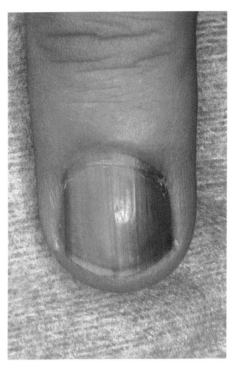

Figure 5.33
Lateral band of longitudinal melanonychia.

longitudinal pigmented streaks within the nail plate (Figures 5.33–5.35). A band of LM may be due to one of four possible mechanisms:

- focal activation of the nail matrix melanocytes
- hyperplasia of the nail matrix melanocytes
- naevus of the nail matrix
- melanoma of the nail matrix.

Table 5.5 lists the causes of LM.

Focal activation of the nail matrix melanocytes

This is the most common cause of LM, and is typified by the presence of melanocytes with

Table 5.5 Causes of longitudinal melanonychia

Racial variation
Laugier–Hunziker–Baran syndrome (Figure 5.34)
Inflammatory nail disorders
Drugs
Irradiation
Fungal
Endocrine diseases
Trauma
Neoplasms
AIDS
Nutritional

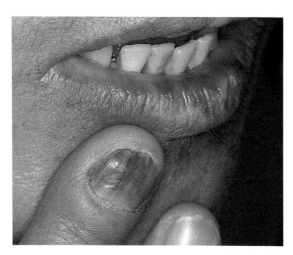

Figure 5.34
Laugier–Hunziker–Baran syndrome – nail and lip hyperpigmentation.

long dendrites located among nail matrix basal layers. There is no atypia or theque formation.

Melanocyte activation occurs in 77% of African-Americans over 20 years of age and in almost 100% of those over 50 years old. It is observed in 10–20% of Japanese individuals as well as in people of Hispanic descent and other dark-skinned groups. It is uncommon in white populations. Normal variant in black population is due to the number and size of melanosomes produced. In white people melanosomes are small and aggregated in complexes. In black people melanosomes are greater in length, larger in diameter and distributed singly within keratinocytes.

Melanocyte activation may be induced by repeated trauma to the nail matrix. Patients who pick, break or chew the skin over the proximal nail fold frequently develop bands of LM. This is usually associated with nail plate surface abnormalities due to repeated nail matrix injury. Frictional LM is commonly observed in the toes of elderly individuals who have foot deformities and/or unsatisfactory footwear. The melanonychia typically appears at the site of friction with the tip of the shoes or under an overriding toe (see Chapter 9). Inflammatory disorders of the nail may also produce nail pigmentation. Post-inflammatory melanonychia has been described in lichen planus, Hallopeau's acrodermatitis and chronic radiodermatitis. *Trichophyton rubrum* and *Scytalidium dimidiatum* (*Hendersonula toruloidea*) nail infection may also occasionally lead to LM. Longitudinal melanonychia may be secondary to the inflammatory changes which induce activation of nail matrix melanocytes, or due to direct melanin production by the fungi.

Activation of nail matrix melanocytes is occasionally seen in endocrine disorders such as Addison's disease, in pregnancy and in patients with human immunodeficiency virus (HIV) infection, even in those not treated with zidovudine (azidothymine, AZT). Nail matrix melanocytes may also be activated by drugs such as AZT, cancer chemotherapeutic agents and psoralens. Drug-induced melanonychia usually involves several digits; it is reversible.

Melanocyte hyperplasia

Melanocyte hyperplasia is characterized by an increased number of melanocytes, which are scattered between nail matrix keratinocytes without 'nest' formation. The pathogenesis of melanocyte hyperplasia is unknown. We have found this pathological picture in patients with a single band of LM. Differential diagnosis from melanoma *in situ* may be difficult, and these bands should be completely excised in order to perform serial sections.

Nail matrix naevus

Congenital and acquired melanocytic naevi may occur in the nail matrix and present as LM. Nail matrix naevi are rare and only a few histologically proven naevi of the nail matrix have been reported. Naevi of the nail matrix are most commonly of the junctional type. The architectural pattern of nail matrix naevi is similar to that of skin naevi. Naevus cells are usually seen arranged in nests at the dermo-epidermal junction. Single naevus cells can sometimes be found among nail matrix basal and suprabasal onychocytes. Dendritic melanocytes are only occasionally present.

Immunostaining with HMB-45 of nail matrix naevi shows a positive reaction in the cells of the epidermal and junctional component as usually seen in acquired skin naevi. Nail pigmentation due to congenital nail matrix melanocytic naevi may spontaneously regress. However, fading of the pigmentation may only relate to decreased activity of the naevus cells rather than regression of the naevus itself.

The frequency of progression from nail matrix naevi to nail matrix melanoma is not known but a few cases have been well documented. Surgical excision of nail matrix naevi is therefore a justified preventive measure.

Malignant melanoma

In the nail apparatus the most common initial sign of melanoma is acquired LM in white

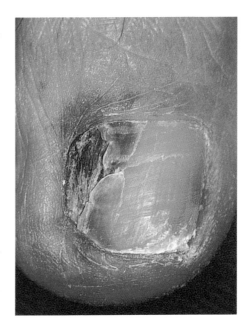

Figure 5.35
Malignant melanoma.

individuals or broadening of an existing band in people of African or Asian descent. This tumour and its practical differential diagnosis from other chromonychias and nail dystrophies is described in this section; linear melanony-chia from other causes is considered in Chapter 7.

Melanoma of the nail region is now better understood since the identification and analysis of acrolentiginous melanoma. It may be localized subungually or periungually with pigmentation and/or dystrophy of the nail plate (Figure 5.35). Initial lesions may be mistaken histologically for benign or atypical melanocytic hyperplasia, but serial sections usually reveal the true nature of the disease.

> **Acquired longitudinal melanonychia after puberty in a white-skinned individual requires urgent biopsy**

Approximately 2–3% of melanomas in whites, and 15–20% in blacks are located in the nail unit. However, malignant melanoma is rare in black people; thus the number of nail melanomas does not significantly differ between these population groups. Most white patients have a fair complexion, light hair, and blue or hazel eyes. There is no sex predominance, although some reports show variable female or male predominance. The mean age at onset is 55–60 years. Most tumours are found in the thumbs or great toes.

Melanoma of the nail region is often asymptomatic. Many patients only notice a pigmented lesion after trauma to the area; only approximately two-thirds seek medical advice because of the appearance of the lesion; pain or discomfort is rare, and nail deformity, spontaneous ulceration, sudden change in colour, bleeding or tumour mass breaking through the nail are even more infrequent. It is useful to remember that a pigmented subungual lesion is more likely to be malignant than benign. If the melanoma is pigmented it may show one or more of the following characteristics:

1 A spot appearing in the matrix, nail bed or plate. This may vary in colour from brown to black; it may be homogeneous or irregular, and is seldom painful.
2 A longitudinal brown to black band of variable width running through the whole visible nail.
3 Less frequently, Hutchinson's sign – periungual extension of brown-black pigmentation from LM onto the proximal and lateral nail folds – is an important indicator of subungual melanoma (but note the reservations discussed below).

Current experience has demonstrated that Hutchinson's sign, while valuable, is not an infallible predictor of melanoma, for the following reasons:

- Periungual pigmentation is present in a variety of benign disorders and, under these circumstances, may lead to overdiagnosis of subungual melanoma.
- Periungual hyperpigmentation occurs in at least one non-melanoma skin cancer: Bowen's disease of the nail unit.
- Hyperpigmentation of the nail bed and matrix may reflect through the 'transparent' nail folds, simulating Hutchinson's sign ('pseudo-Hutchinson's sign'). Each of the above may incorrectly suggest a diagnosis of subungual melanoma. Table 5.6 lists disorders in which pseudo-Hutchinson's sign occurs.

Total reliance on the (apparent) presence or absence of periungual pigmentation may lead to over- or underdiagnosis of subungual melanoma. All relevant clinical and historical information, including the presence or absence of periungual pigmentation, must be carefully evaluated in a patient suspected of having subungual melanoma. Ultimately, the diagnosis of subungual melanoma is made histologically. Hutchinson's sign is a single, important clue to this diagnosis. The nail plate may also become thickened or fissured and permanently shed.

Approximately 25% of melanomas are amelanotic (pigmentation not an obvious or prominent sign; Figure 5.36) and may mimic pyogenic granuloma, granulation tissue or ingrowing nail. The risk of misdiagnosis is particularly high in these cases.

Malignant melanoma must be considered in the differential diagnosis (see Table 5.3) in all cases of inexplicable chronic paronychia, whether painful or not, in torpid granulomatous ulceration of the proximal nail fold and in pseudoverrucous keratotic lesions of the nail bed and lateral nail groove. Subungual melanoma may also simulate mycobacterial infections, mycotic onychodystrophy, recalcitrant paronychia and ingrowing nail. Subungual haematoma is not rare and may present

Table 5.6 Disorders accompanied by pseudo-Hutchinson's sign

Disorder	Clinical features
Benign	
Illusory pigmentation	Dark colour is visible because of the cuticle and thin nail fold transparency and not because of melanin localization within these tissues
Ethnic pigmentation	Proximal nail fold of dark-skinned persons – lateral nail folds not involved; LM may be present or absent; often exaggerated in thumbs
Naevoid lentigo	May recur after surgical removal
Laugier–Hunziker–Baran syndrome	Macular pigmentation of lips, mouth and genitalia; one or several fingers involved
Peutz–Jeghers syndrome	Hyperpigmentation of fingers and toes, macular pigmentation of buccal mucosa and lips
Addison's disease	Diffuse tanning of both exposed and non-exposed portions of the body; bluish-black discoloration of the mucous membranes of the lips and mouth
X-ray therapy	Treatment for finger dermatitis, psoriasis and chronic paronychia
Malnutrition	Polydactylous involvement
Minocycline	Polydactylous involvement
AIDS patients	Polydactylous involvement; zidovudine produces similar features
Trauma	Due to friction, nail biting and picking, or boxing
Congenital or acquired naevus after biopsy	Pigment recurrence after biopsy of LM in acquired and congenital melanocytic naevi, often striking cytologic atypia
Regressing naevoid melanosis in childhood	Monodactylous; initial increase in dyschromia followed by subsequent pigment regression; perplexing disorder
Subungual haematoma	Exceptionally, blood spreads to nail folds and the hyponychial area
Silver nitrate	For treatment of granulation tissue; may produce a black halo
Malignant	
Bowen's disease	Features clinically typical of subungual melanoma

(After Baran and Kichijian (1996).
LM, longitudinal melanonychia.

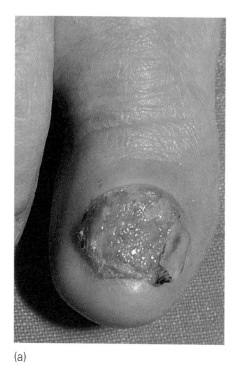

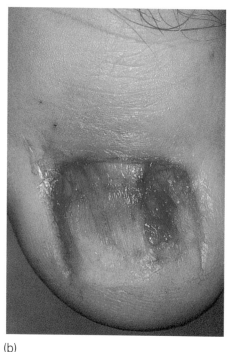

Figure 5.36
(a, b) Malignant melanoma – amelanotic.

(a)   (b)

without a history of severe trauma. It may follow repeated minor trauma which escapes the patient's attention, such as in 'tennis toe', or follow trauma from wearing hard ski boots. Although haematoma following a single traumatic event usually grows out in one piece, rather than as a longitudinal streak due to the continuous production of pigment, repeated trauma may cause difficulties in differential diagnosis. It is recommended that the lesion should be examined with a magnifying loupe after it has been covered with a drop of oil. The pigmented nail should be clipped and tested with the argentaffin reaction in order to rule out melanin pigmentation. Subungual haemoglobin is not degraded to haemosiderin and is therefore negative to staining with Prussian blue. Scrapings or small pieces of the nail boiled with water in a test tube give a positive benzidine reaction with the conventional haemoglobin reagent strips. The difference between haemosiderinic and melanotic pigment, sometimes difficult to discern by routine histological methods, is easily seen by ultrastructural techniques: ferrous pigment is intercellular while melanin is intracellular.

Because of its frequency, melanonychia striata in people with deeply pigmented skin is considered a normal finding, but up to one-fifth of all melanomas in black patients are in the subungual area, and these typically begin with a pigmented spot producing a longitudinal streak. These spots are usually black rather than the normal brown. The diagnosis may be aided by comparing them with the brown stripes in other nails or by the occurrence of Hutchinson's sign.

The following guidelines should be adhered to where possible to enable accurate tissue diagnosis to be made and appropriate treatment carried out. As a first step, the anatomical site of the matrix affected will be obtained from the level of the melanin pigment identified with Fontana's silver stain of a nail clipping obtained from the distal free edge. The type of biopsy selected will then depend on the site of the matrix melanin production, the width of the linear pigmentation, and the site of the band in the nail plate. If the pigment is located within the ventral portion of the nail plate, a decision has to be made depending on the width of the band:

- A punch biopsy should be used when the width of the band is less than 3 mm. If the base of the nail plate is removed, the specimen may be released more easily, and the integrity of the region distal to the biopsied matrix area may be checked.
- A transverse matrix biopsy should be used for a band wider than 3 mm.

If the pigment involves the upper portion of the nail, it is obviously difficult to use the two previous procedures to remove the source of melanin pigment, for anatomical reasons and because of the risk of a secondary dystrophy, thus:

- A rectangular block of tissue is excised using two parallel incisions down to the bone. An L-shaped incision is carried back along the lateral nail wall, freeing this flap. The lateral section may then be rotated medially and approximated to the remaining nail segment.
- If the band is wider than 6 mm or if the whole thickness of the nail is involved by the pigment, surgical removal of the nail apparatus seems the most logical method. However, one (or even two) 3 mm punch biopsy is an alternative prior to more radical treatment, especially in young women.
- When the band lies within the lateral third of the nail plate, lateral longitudinal biopsy is more suitable.
- If LM is accompanied by periungual pigmentation (Hutchinson's sign), removal of the nail apparatus is required.

Histological examination of acral lentiginous melanoma requires great experience, and often serial sections are needed to classify the lesion accurately. Grading according to Clark's levels or Breslow's maximum tumour thickness is difficult and often inconclusive.

> **Nail apparatus melanoma has a poor prognosis, with up to 50% of patients dying within 5 years of the diagnosis**

Subungual melanoma has a poor prognosis. The reported 5-year survival rates range from 35% to 50%. Most patients present with advanced subungual melanoma; however, even early diagnosis is not a guarantee of a good prognosis. Women have a better prognosis than men. Factors contributing to a poor prognosis are delay in diagnosis and, as a result of this, inadequate treatment. The tumour may be mistaken for a traumatic dystrophy, and valuable time may be lost before the diagnosis is made.

Treatment depends on the stage of the disease. Levels I and II melanomas may be adequately treated by wide local excision, and repair of the defect with graft or flap. Amputation is usually advised for melanoma at levels more advanced than II. When the thumb has to be amputated, pollicization of a finger may provide a functional replacement. There would appear to be no relationship between the prognosis and the extent of the amputation, although metacarpo/metatarsophalangeal amputation is considered to be inadequate because of local recurrences. The rationale for elective lymph node dissection and/or isolated hyperthermic perfusion of the extremity with cytotoxic drugs is still under discussion. Immune enhancement such as BCG (bacillus Calmette–Guérin) therapy is used in some centres.

Table 5.7 Conditions in which nail pustulation may occur

Infective (primary cause)
    Acute paronychia (see p. 81)
    Blistering distal dactylitis
    Hand, foot and mouth disease
    Herpes simplex (primary and recurrent)
    Gonorrhoea
    Impetigo
    Veillonella infection (in newborns)

Non-infective (secondary infection may occur)
    Ingrowing toe nail
        Malalignment in childhood
        Common type
    Self-inflicted bullous lesions of newborn
    Thumb sucking (and paronychia)

Dermatoses
    Acrokeratosis paraneoplastica
    Acropustulosis/psoriasis
    Parakeratosis pustulosa
    Reiter's syndrome

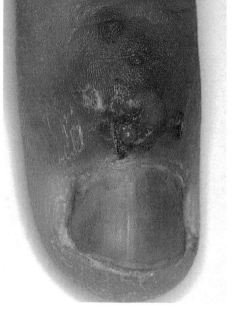

Figure 5.37
Primary herpes simplex – herpetic 'whitlow'.

PUSTULES

The conditions in which nail apparatus pustulation may be a significant sign are listed in Table 5.7.

Herpes simplex

Distal digital herpes simplex infection may affect the terminal phalanx as a primary herpetic 'whitlow' or start as an acute, intensely painful paronychia (Figures 5.37, 5.38). It is relatively common in dental staff, anaesthetists and those involved with the care of the mouth and upper respiratory tract in unconscious patients. Recurrent forms are

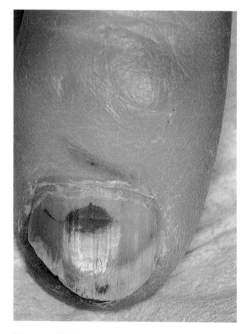

Figure 5.38
Subungual recurrent herpes simplex.

generally less severe and have a milder clinical course than the initial infection.

After an incubation period of 3–7 days, during which local tenderness, erythema and swelling may develop, a crop of vesicles appears at the site of origin in the skin. The vesicles are typically distributed in the paronychia and on the volar digital skin, resembling pyogenic infection of the finger tip. Close inspection, however, will reveal the characteristic pale, raised vesicles surrounded by an erythematous border. An acutely painful whitlow may develop and extend under the distal free edge of the nail and into the nail bed. A distinct predilection for the thumb, index and ring fingers on the dominant hand has been noted, but any finger may be involved. Multiple lesions are rare. For 10–14 days the vesicles gradually increase in size, often coalescing into large, honeycombed bullae. New crops of lesions may appear during this time. Vesicular fluid is clear early in the disease but may become turbid, seropurulent or even haemorrhagic within days of onset. At times, a pale yellow colour of the vesicles will suggest pyogenic infection, yet frank pus is not usually obtained. Patients complain of tenderness and severe throbbing in the affected digit. Coexisting primary herpetic infections of the mouth and finger nails suggest auto-inoculation of the virus into the nail tissues as a result of nail biting or finger sucking.

Radiating pain along the C7 spinal nerve distribution is sometimes noted before each recurrence. Lymphangitis may start from the wrist and extend to the axilla with painful lymphadenopathy. Numbness and hypo-aesthesia following the acute episode have been observed.

The diagnosis of herpetic infection can be made by examining the base of the vesicles for the characteristic multinucleated 'balloon' giant cells, in stained smears. The presence of intranuclear inclusions is also significant. Viral cultivation, usually positive within 24 hours of onset, is confirmatory; the active viral phase lasts up to 4–5 days in primary attacks but only 2–3 days in recurrent episodes.

Differential diagnosis

It is important to exclude primary or recurrent herpes simplex infection in the differential diagnosis of every vesiculopustular finger infection. The typical appearance of the lesions with disproportionately severe pain, the absence of pus in the confluent, multiloculated, vesiculopustular lesions and the lack of increased tension in the finger pulp aid in differentiating this slow-healing infection from a bacterial foreign body or paronychia.

Herpes zoster infections, which may affect the proximal nail fold like herpes simplex, also involve the entire sensory dermatome. The pustules of primary cutaneous *Neisseria gonorrhoeae* infection may resemble herpes simplex on the rare occasion when it occurs on the finger. The diagnosis is established by positive Gram staining and bacteriological culture.

Treatment

Treatment is aimed primarily at symptomatic relief and the avoidance of secondary infection. Topical acyclovir may shorten the course of any one attack; given orally the drug may prevent recurrences while it is being taken. On cessation of the treatment relapses are unfortunately common. This is a preventable infection. Gloves should always be worn on both hands for procedures such as intubation, removal of dentures or providing oral care, despite the additional costs involved.

Veillonella infection in the newborn

Many epidemics of subungual infection have been described among infants in postnatal wards and special care baby units. The number of fingers affected per patient ranged from one to ten; the thumbs are less frequently involved than other fingers; toe nails are not affected. Three stages occur: first, a small amount of clear fluid appears under the centre of the nail, along with mild inflammation at the distal end of the finger. This initial vesicle lasts approximately 24 hours; it sometimes enlarges but never extends to the edge of the nail. Some small lesions bypass the second, pustular stage, going directly to the third stage. As a rule the fluid becomes yellow after 24 hours, the pus remaining for 24–48 hours, before gradually turning brown and being absorbed. The colour fades progressively over a period of 2–6 weeks, leaving the nail and nail bed completely normal.

Subungual pus obtained by aseptic puncture of the nails shows tiny, Gram-negative cocci about 0.4 μm in diameter. These organisms resemble *Veillonella*, a group of anaerobes of dubious pathogenicity found as commensals in the saliva, vagina and respiratory tract. Systemic antibiotics do not change the clinical course of the nail lesions, which do not differ from those observed in other untreated and affected newborn children.

Impetigo

The dorsal aspect of the distal phalanx may be involved by impetigo (Figure 5.39). It presents in two forms:

1 Vesiculopustular, with its familiar honey-crusted lesions, usually due to beta-haemolytic streptococci.
2 Bullous, usually due to phage type 71 staphylococci.

The latter is characterized by the appearance of large, localized, intra-epidermal bullae that persist for longer periods than the transient vesicles of streptococcal impetigo which subsequently rupture spontaneously to form very thin crusts. The lesions of bullous impetigo may mimic the non-infectious bullous diseases (such as drug-induced types or pemphigoid). Oral therapy of bullous impetigo with a penicillinase-resistant penicillin should be instituted and continued until the lesions resolve. Cephalexin and erythromycin are acceptable alternatives. The lesions should be cleansed several times daily and topical aureomycin (3%) applied to all the affected areas.

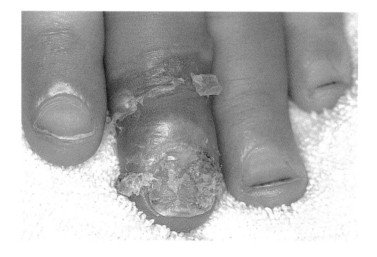

Figure 5.39
Impetigo of the nail apparatus.

Blistering distal dactylitis

Blistering distal dactylitis is a variant of streptococcal skin infection. It presents as a superficial, tender, blistering beta-haemolytic streptococcal infection over the anterior fat pad of the distal phalanx of the finger (Figure 5.40). The lesion may or may not have a paronychial extension. This blister, containing thin, white pus, has a predilection for the tip of the digit and extends to the subungual area of the free edge of the nail plate. The area may provide a nidus for the beta-haemolytic streptococcus and act as a focus of chronic infection similar to the nasopharynx. The age range of affected patients is 2–16 years. For local care incision, drainage and antiseptic soaking are indicated, giving a more rapid response than systemic antibiotic therapy alone: effective regimens include benzylpenicillin (penicillin G) in a single intramuscular dose, a 10-day course of oral phenoxymethylpenicillin or eryhromycin ethyl succinate. This type of treatment decreases the reservoir of streptococci by preventing spread to family contacts. This infection has been described as a complication of ingrowing toe nail. The differential diagnosis includes blisters resulting from friction, thermal and chemical burns, infectious states such as herpetic whitlow, staphylococcal bullous impetigo and the Weber–Cockayne variant of epidermolysis bullosa simplex.

Chronic paronychia and thumb sucking

Candidal paronychia, usually in association with oral candidiasis, may arise as a result of chronic maceration due to thumb sucking (Figure 5.41). Chronic paronychia is not uncommon in children. It differs from the condition seen in adults in the source of the maceration, associated diseases, the clinical appearances of the lesion, and the patient's responses to the symptoms. In children the lesions are generally prominent, with total

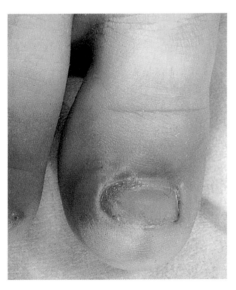

Figure 5.40
Blistering distal dactylitis.

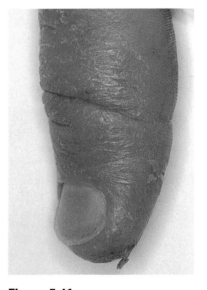

Figure 5.41
Chronic paronychia caused by thumb sucking in an atopic individual.

involvement of the proximal nail fold. The skin is usually erythematous and glistening owing to the wet environment produced by continuous thumb sucking. The quality of the nail is always altered, resulting in a poor texture. The habit of sucking fingers or thumbs is the most important predisposing factor. *Candida albicans* is present in all cases. When an acute flare-up occurs the patient experiences pruritus and discomfort in the proximal nail fold. Children respond to this by sucking – the symptoms of chronic paronychia perpetuating the habit that initiated the maceration. The lesions tend to be more severe in childhood than in adult paronychia, probably because thumb sucking is more continuous than exposure to wet work, and saliva is more irritating than water. The minor repeated trauma resulting from suction is capable of causing complete loss of the nail plate. Detection of the carrier state in the mouth and gastrointestinal tract by cultures of saliva and stools may be important in the occasional patient with refractory paronychia. Persistent and repeated candidal paronychia in infancy suggests a more serious underlying disorder and such infants should be investigated for endocrine disease and immune deficiency syndromes.

Thumb or finger sucking is sometimes associated with herpes simplex. This may result in local extension of the eruption producing viral stomatitis combined with involvement of the digit. In childhood, local trauma, caused by onychophagia, may result in the development of opportunistic infection by the normal oropharyngeal flora, amongst which are found HB 1 bacteria. Acute paronychia may also be caused by HB 1 organisms (*Eikenella corrodens*), but this is uncommon in the absence of immune deficiency.

Acropustulosis and pustular psoriasis

In pustular psoriasis and acrodermatitis continua (Hallopeau's disease), involvement of a single digit is common. It is often misdiagnosed when the pustule appears beneath the nail plate with necrosis of tissue resulting in desiccation and crust formation. New pustule formation may develop at the periphery or within the lesions. The nail is lifted off by the crust and lakes of pus and new pustules may form on the denuded nail bed (Figures 5.42–5.44). Permanent loss is possible. Acral pustular psoriasis has been reported with resorptive osteolysis ('deep Koebner phenomenon') and pronounced skin and subcutaneous tissue atrophy. There may be progressive loss of entire digits in the feet and loss of finger tips and finger nails. 'Tuft' osteolysis may occur independently of acropustuloses and arthritis. Histopathology reveals Munro–Sabouraud 'micro-abscesses' or the spongiform pustule of Kogoj. Localized psoralens with ultraviolet irradication (PUVA) therapy can be of benefit. Oral retinoid therapy may give good short-term results, but recurrences appear 1–3 months after the treatment has been stopped. Combined retinoid and PUVA treatment delays

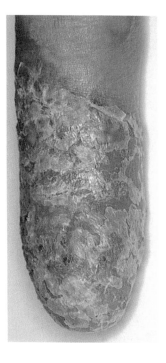

Figure 5.42 Psoriatic acropustulosis (Hallopeau's disease).

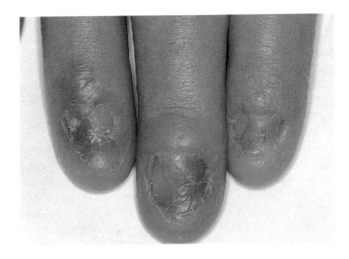

Figure 5.43
Pustular psoriasis.

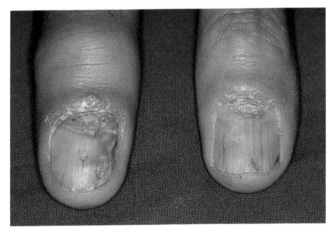

Figure 5.44
Proximal nail fold pustular psoriasis –
limited form of acropustulosis.

and lowers the frequency of relapses. Topical mechlorethamine has given some good results, as has intramuscular triamcinolone acetonide.

The differential diagnosis of acropustulosis may be controversial, particularly with regard to the subcorneal pustular dermatosis of Sneddon and Wilkinson. Many authorities have described patients with pustular lesions like those described as subcorneal pustular dermatosis, but who had in addition stigmata suggestive of psoriasis. These included typical scaly plaques on the elbows and knees, pitted nails or arthropathy. It is, however, pointless to debate the pathogenesis of Sneddon–Wilkinson disease

without applying the techniques available for identifying the psoriatic state: cell kinetics, complement activation in the stratum corneum, human leucocyte antigen (HLA) family studies and nail growth studies.

Reiter's syndrome

The clinical and histological features of the skin changes in Reiter's syndrome may be indistinguishable from those of psoriasis. Skin changes resembling paronychia can accompany nail

All the nail signs in Reiter's syndrome
may be present in severe psoriasis

involvement, suggesting inflammation of the proximal nail fold. Onycholysis, ridging, splitting, greenish-yellow or sometimes brownish-red discoloration and subungual hyperkeratosis may be present. Small yellow pustules may develop and slowly enlarge beneath the nail, often near the lunula. Their contents become dry and brown. The nails may be shed. Nail pitting may be seen in Reiter's syndrome, individual pits being deep and punched out. This nail pitting may reflect a predisposition to the development of psoriasis or psoriasiform lesions dependent on the HLA-A2 and B27 antigens, as suggested by previously reported HLA typing studies. Both HLA-A2 and B27 were present in a 6–year-old boy who had only the nail changes which were compatible with Reiter's syndrome; the same antigens were also present in his father, who had uveitis, arthritis and amyloidosis.

Antibiotics, steroids and non-steroidal anti-inflammatory drugs are without benefit; PUVA may be helpful. Oral retinoid therapy may clear the nails in Reiter's syndrome. Combined chemotherapy with methotrexate, oral retinoid and prednisolone has been suggested.

Parakeratosis pustulosa (Hjorth–Sabouraud syndrome)

This parakeratotic condition of the finger tip was first described more than 50 years ago. It usually occurs in girls of approximately 7 years of age, typically affecting only one digit, usually a finger (Figure 5.45). The lesions start close to the free margin of the nail of a finger or toe. In some cases, a few isolated pustules or vesicles may be observed in the initial phase;

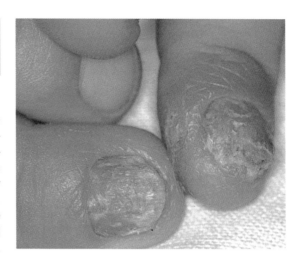

Figure 5.45
Parakeratosis pustulosa.

these usually disappear before the patient presents to the doctor. Confluent eczematoid changes cover the skin immediately adjacent to the distal edge of the nail. The affected area is pink or of normal skin colour and densely studded with fine scales; there is a clear margin between the normal and affected areas. The skin changes may extend to the dorsal aspect of the finger or toe, but usually only the finger tip is affected. The most striking and characteristic change is the hyperkeratosis beneath the nail tip. The nail plate is lifted up, deformed and often thickened. Commonly the deformity produced is asymmetrical and limited to one corner of the distal edge, or at least more pronounced at the corners of the nail. Pitting occurs in some cases; rarely, transverse ridging of the nail plate is present. In most cases the condition resolves within a few months, but in some cases it may persist for many years, even into adult life.

Histological findings are of some value, including hyperkeratosis and parakeratosis, pustulation and crusts, acanthosis and mild exocytosis, papillomatosis and heavy cellular infiltrates composed mainly of lymphocytes and fibroblasts around dilated capillary loops. This histological picture presents many of the features common to psoriasis and eczema.

In the differential diagnosis of parakeratosis pustulosa, the following points are important:

- Pustules are rare and are only seen in the initial stage, unlike pustular psoriasis or acropustulosis.
- Patients with psoriasis develop a coarse sheet of scales and not the fine type of scaling typically seen in parakeratosis pustulosa.
- If the nail changes predominate, especially on a toe, the disorder can be mistaken for onychomycosis. Thumb sucking, which is a predisposing factor in chronic candidal paronychia, should be ruled out when a single thumb is affected.

No treatment makes any difference to the frequency of recurrence or the overall duration of parakeratosis pustulosa. Topical steroids provide some symptomatic relief.

Acrokeratosis paraneoplastica of Bazex and Dupré

Acrokeratosis paraneoplastica occurs in association with malignant epithelial tumours of the upper respiratory or digestive tracts, in particular the pharyngolaryngeal area piriform fossa, tonsillar area, epiglottis, hard and soft palate, vocal cords, tongue, lower lip, oesophagus and the upper third of the lungs. It also occurs with metastases to the cervical and upper mediastinal lymph nodes. This 'paraneoplasia' may precede the signs of the associated malignancy, disappear when the tumour is removed and reappear with its recurrence; however, the nail involvement does not always benefit from total recovery, in contrast to the other lesions. This condition almost exclusively occurs in men over 40 years of age. The lesions are erythematous, violaceous and keratotic with ill-defined borders. They are symmetrically distributed, affecting hands, feet, ears and occasionally the nose. The toe nails suffer more severely than the finger nails. Roughened, irregular, keratotic, fissured and warty excrescences are found equally on the terminal phalanges of both fingers and toes (Figure 5.46).

The nails are invariably involved and are typically the earliest manifestation of the disease. In mild forms, the nail involvement is discrete; the affected nails are thin and soft, and may become fragile and crumble. In more established disease, the nails are flaky, irregular and whitened, and the free edge is raised by subungual hyperkeratosis. In severe forms, the

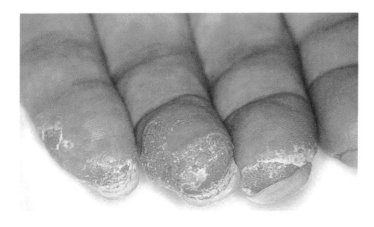

Figure 5.46
Psoriasis-like Acrokeratosis paraneoplastica.

lesions resemble advanced psoriatic nail dystrophy and may progress to complete loss of the diseased nails. The nail bed is eventually replaced by a smooth epidermis to which the irregular, horny vestiges of the nail still adhere. The periungual skin shows an erythemato-squamous eruption, predominantly on the dorsum of the terminal phalanges; there may be associated chronic paronychia with occasional acute suppurative exacerbations.

The two extremes of the disease may coexist. In these cases, the proximal third of the nail is atrophic and the distal two-thirds exhibits hypertrophic changes. The histopathological changes are non-specific, although they do enable the exclusion of a diagnosis of psoriasis, lupus erythematosus or other similar eruptions.

MISCELLANEOUS DERMATOSES

Virtually all skin diseases can sometimes affect the paronychial tissue. It is therefore wise to examine the entire skin of a patient presenting with lesions of the periungual skin.

FURTHER READING

Paronychia

Baran R, Bureau H (1983) Congenital malalignment of the big toe-nail as a cause of ingrowing toe-nail in infancy. Pathology and treatment (a study of thirty cases), *Clin Exp Dermatol* **8**: 619–623.

Barth JH, Dawber RPR (1987) Diseases of the nails in children, *Pediatr Dermatol* **4**: 275–290.

Editorial (1975) Chronic paronychia, *BMJ* **ii**: 460.

Stone OJ, Mullins JF, Head ES (1964) Chronic paronychia. Occupational material, *Arch Environ Health* **9**: 585–588.

Stone OJ, Mullins FJ (1968) Chronic paronychia in children, *Clin Pediatr* **7**: 104–107.

Tosti A, Guerra L, Morelli R, Bardazzi F, Fanti PA (1992) Role of foods in the pathogenesis of chronic paronychia, *J Am Acad Dermatol* **27**: 706–710.

Zaias N (1990) *The Nail in Health and Disease*, 2nd edn (Appleton & Lange, East Norwalk).

Tumours and swellings

Baran R, Kichijian P (1989) Longitudinal melanonychia. Diagnosis and management, *J Am Acad Dermatol* **21**: 1165–1175.

Baran R, Kichijian P (1996) Hutchinson's sign: a reappraisal, *J Am Acad Dermatol* **34**: 87–90.

Briggs JC (1985) Subungual malignant melanoma: a review article, *Br J Plast Surg* **38**: 174–176.

Salasche SJ, Garland LD (1985) Tumours of the nail, *Dermatol Clin* **3**: 501–519.

Pustules

Hjorth N, Thomsen K (1967) Parakeratosis pustulosa, *Br J Dermatol* **79**: 527–532.

6 Nail consistency

Robert Baran, Rodney PR Dawber, Eckart Haneke, Antonella Tosti

Hard nails • Fragile, brittle and soft nails

HARD NAILS

Hard nails are not uncommon on the toes, where they may present as onychogryphosis. In contrast, hard finger nails are unusual and are principally observed in an ectodermal dysplasia, pachyonychia congenita. The nails become yellowish-brown usually within months after birth and show subungual hyperkeratosis with elevation of the nail plate. The nails become progressively thicker and wedge-shaped. Jadassohn had to use a hammer and chisel on the hardened nails of his patient.

Nail hardness is one of the most conspicuous sign of the triad of yellow nail syndrome. They are associated with a very slow growth rate. The nails are thickened with increased transverse curvature; hardness of the nails (scleronychia syndrome) makes it difficult to take a biopsy through the nail plate.

FRAGILE, BRITTLE AND SOFT NAILS

Many of the nail diseases that disrupt nail formation and structure cause secondary brittleness and fragility. In this chapter only those conditions leading to nail fragility or brittleness as a major sign are considered in any detail (Figures 6.1–6.7).

'Hapalonychia' is the term used for cryptogenic soft nail – cases for which there is no primary specific local nail disease to explain the change. Diseases and conditions associated with this include:

* congenital types
* sulphur deficiency syndromes

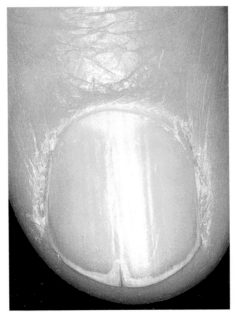

Figure 6.1
Distal nail fissure.

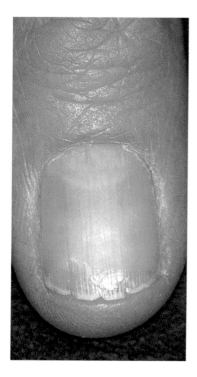

Figure 6.2
Distal nail fragility. Crenellated distal splitting associated with distal onycho-schizia (splitting into layers).

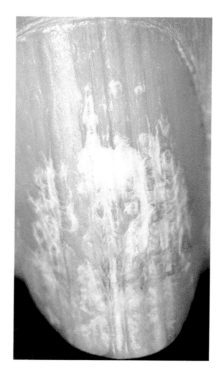

Figure 6.3
Surface nail fragility and fractures due to nail varnish (keratin granulations).

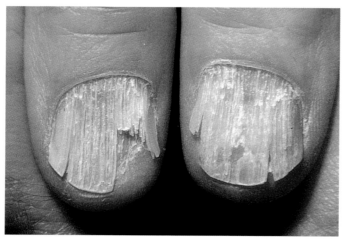

Figure 6.4
Nail fragility in lichen planus. (ridging, splitting and onychoschizia).

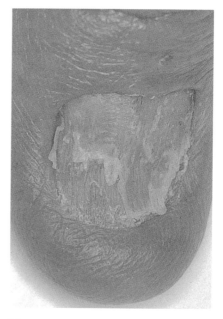

Figure 6.5
Severe nail plate fragility after etretinate therapy before loss.

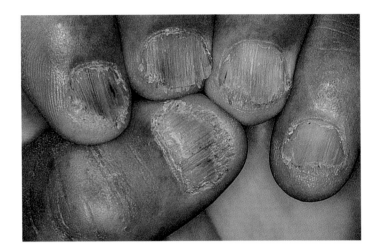

Figure 6.6
Nail apparatus – amyloidosis.

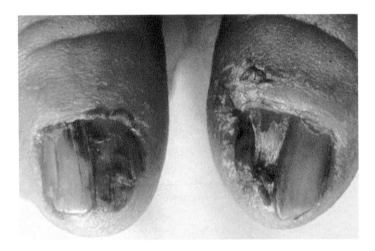

Figure 6.7
Darier's disease, with some nail plate loss.

- thin nail plate of any cause
- occupational disease (for example working with industrial oils)
- chronic arthritis
- leprosy
- hypothyroidism
- peripheral ischaemia
- peripheral neuritis
- hemiplegia
- cachexic states.

In some cases of hapalonychia the thinned nails assumed a semi-transparent, bluish-white hue, sometimes described as 'eggshell nails'.

Nail fragility syndrome can be divided into six main types on morphological grounds:

1   An isolated longitudinal split at the free edge which sometimes extends proximally.
2   This may result from onychorrhexis with shallow parallel furrows running on the superficial layer of the nail.
3   Multiple, crenellated splitting which resembles the battlements of a castle. Triangular pieces may easily be torn from the free margin.

4 Lamellar splitting of the free edge of the nail into horizontal fine layers (onychoschizia) (see Figures 3.39, 3.43). This may occur alone or associated with the other types.

5 Transverse splitting and breaking of the lateral edge close to the distal margin.

6 Nail friability is observed in psoriasis, onychomycosis and as adverse effect of nail varnish (keratin granulations, figure 6.3).

The changes in brittle, friable nails are often confined to the surface of the nail plate; this occurs in superficial white onychomycosis and may be seen after the application of nail polish or base coat which causes 'granulations' in the nail keratin. In advanced psoriasis and fungal infection the friability may extend throughout the entire nail.

The changes in nail consistency may be due to impairment of one or more of the factors on which the health of the nail depends, for example variations in the water content or keratin structure and corneocyte adhesion. In addition, changes in the intercellular structures and cell membranes, and intracellular changes in the arrangement of keratin fibrils, have been revealed by electron microscopy. Normal nails contain approximately 18% water. After prolonged immersion in water this percentage is increased and the nail becomes soft; this makes toe-nail trimming and nail biopsies much easier. A low lipid content may decrease the nail's ability to retain water. If the water content is considerably reduced, the nail becomes brittle. Splitting, which results from this brittle quality, is probably partly due to repeated uptake and rapid drying out.

The keratin content may be modified by chemical and physical insults, especially in occupational nail disorders. Amino acid chains may be broken or distorted by alkalis, oxidizing agents and thioglycollates (used in the permanent waving of hair). These break or distort the multiple disulphide bond linkages which join

Table 6.1 Factors leading to fragile, brittle or soft nails

Local factors
  Trauma
    Occupational
    Onychotillomania
  Chemical

Dermatological conditions (may thin the nail plate)
  Alopecia areata
  Amyloidosis
  Darier's disease
  Eczema
  Lichen planus
  Lichen striatus
  Onychomycosis
  Psoriasis
  Slow nail growth

General factors
  Aging (fingers)
  Anaemia (iron deficiency)
  Cachexic state
  Chronic arthropathies (fingers or toes)
  Drugs
    Antimetabolites
    Arsenic
    Acitretine (etretinate)
    Gold salts
    Penicillamine
  Vitamin A, C and B_6 deficiencies
  Gout
  Graft-versus-host disease
  Haemodialysis
  Hyper- or hypothyroidism
  Neurological
    Hemiplegia
    Neuropathies
  Osteomalacia
  Osteoporosis
  Peripheral circulatory impairment (arterial)
  Pregnancy
  Sulphur deficiency diseases

the protein chains to form the keratin fibrils. Keratin structure can also be changed in genetic disorders such as dyskeratosis congenita, in which the nail plate is completely absent or reduced to thin, dystrophic remnants. The composition of the nail plate is sometimes related to generalized disease. A high sulphur content, predominantly in the form of cystine, contributes to the stability of the fibrous protein by the formation of disulphide bonds. A lack of iron can result in softening of the nail and koilonychia; conversely, the calcium content of the nail appears to contribute little towards its hardness. Age-dependant decrease in cholesterol sulfate levels might explain the higher incidence of brittle nails in women. Calcium is located mainly in the surface of the nail, in small absorbed quantities, and X-ray diffraction shows no evidence of calcite or apatite crystals.

Damage to either the central or the peripheral nervous system may result in nail fragility.

factors may affect the hydration of the nail plate.

Fragility, due to thinning of the nail plate, may be caused by a reduction in the length of the matrix. Diminution or even complete arrest of nail formation over a variable width may be the result of many dermatoses such as eczema, lichen planus, psoriasis (rare) and impairment of the peripheral circulation. The frequency of nail fragility in alopecia areata lends credence to the popular belief that nail and hair disorders are often associated.

General causes

General causes of nail fragility are listed in Table 6.1. The diverse constituents of the nail plate, especially the enzymes necessary for the formation of keratin, are subject to genetic influences; changes in these are exhibited in the form of hereditary disease.

Local causes

The nail may be damaged by repeated trauma or by chemical agents such as detergents, alkalis, various solvents, sugar solutions and especially by hot water. The nail plate takes a minimum of 5–6 months to regenerate and therefore it is vulnerable to daily insults. Housework is commonly the cause; particularly at risk are the first three fingers of the dominant hand. Anything that slows the rate of nail growth will increase the risk. Cosmetic causes are rare. Some varnishes will damage the superficial layers of the nail. Drying may be enhanced by some nail varnish removers. Soaking fingers in warm soapy solution, for removing the cuticle, is especially dangerous; this is common practice among manicurists. It has been shown that climatic and seasonal

FURTHER READING

Finlay AY, Frost P, Keith AD et al. An assessment of factors influencing flexibility of human fingernails. *Br J. Dermatol* 1980; **103**: 357–365.

Flowersheim GL. Behandlung brüchiger fingernägels mit biotin. *Zschr Hautkr* 1991; **64**: 31–48.

Lubach D, Beckers P. Wet working conditions increases brittleness of nails, but do not cause it. *Dermatology* 1992; **185**: 120–122.

Saniman P. Nail disorders caused by external influences *J Soc Cosm Chem* 1977; **28**: 351–356.

Brosch T, Pressler S, Platt D. Age-associated changes in integral cholesterol and cholesterol sulfate concentrations in human scalp hair and fingernail clippings. *Aging Clin Exp Res* 2001; **13**: 131–138.

7 Nail colour changes (chromonychia)

Eckart Haneke, Robert Baran, Rodney PR Dawber, Antonella Tosti

Leukonychia (white nail) • Melanonychia (brown or black nail) • Other discolorations • Further reading

The term 'chromonychia' indicates an abnormality in colour of the substance or the surface of the nail plate and/or subungual tissues. Generally, abnormalities of colour depend on the transparency of the nail, its attachments and the character of the underlying tissues. Pigment may accumulate due to overproduction (melanin) or storage (haemosiderin, copper, various drugs), or by surface deposition. The nails provide a historical record for up to 2 years (depending on the rate of linear nail growth) of profound temporary abnormalities of the control of skin pigment which otherwise might pass unnoticed. Colour is also affected by the state of the skin vessels, and by various intravascular factors such as anaemia and carbon monoxide poisoning.

There are some important points to note concerning the examination of abnormal nails for colour changes. The nails should be studied with the fingers completely relaxed and not pressed against any surface. Failure to do this alters the haemodynamics of the nail and changes its appearance. The finger tips should then be blanched by pressing them on an even surface to see if the nail bed is grossly altered; this may help to differentiate between discoloration of the nail plate and its vascular bed. If the discoloration is in the vascular bed, it will usually disappear. Further information can be gleaned by transillumination (diaphanoscopy)

> **Complex internal diseases may sometimes be diagnosed solely by colour changes in the nail apparatus**

of the nail using a pen torch placed against the pulp. If the discoloration is in the matrix or soft tissue, the exact position can be identified more easily and dark material or a non-transparent foreign body will give a dark shadow. Furthermore, if a topical agent or superficial infection is suspected as the cause, one can remove the discoloration by scraping or cleaning the nail plate with a solvent such as acetone. If the substance is impregnated more deeply into the nail or subungually, microscopic studies of potassium hydroxide preparations, tangential or punch biopsy specimens using special stains may be indicated. Wood's lamp examination is sometimes useful.

When the discoloration is of exogenous origin, for example from nail contact with occupationally derived agents or topical application of therapeutic agents, the discoloration typically follows the contour of the proximal nail fold when the discoloured nail grows out. If the proximal margin of the discoloration corresponds to the shape of the lunula an internal cause is likely.

LEUKONYCHIA (WHITE NAIL)

White nails are the most common form of colour change. These can be divided into the following main types:

1 True leukonychia, in which the nail plate is involved.
2 Apparent leukonychia, with involvement of the subungual tissue.
3 Pseudoleukonychia.

In true leukonychia (Figure 7.1) the nail appears opaque and white, probably owing to the diffraction of light in the abnormal keratotic cells; with polarized light, the nail structure appears disrupted owing to disorganization of the keratin fibrils. Total leukonychia, in which the entire nail is affected, is rare. Subtotal leukonychia with incomplete nail plate involvement is more frequent. These forms can be temporary or permanent depending on their aetiology. Partial forms are divided into punctate leukonychia, which is common; striate leukonychia, which is relatively common; and distal leukonychia, which is rare. The term 'pseudoleukonychia' is used when fungal infection involves the nail plate, for example in superficial white onychomycoses, or when nail varnish produces keratin granulation. Apparent leukonychia can be further subdivided into a white appearance of the nail due to:

• underlying onycholysis and subungual hyperkeratosis
• modification of the matrix and/or the nail bed, giving rise, for example, to apparent macrolunula.

True leukonychia

Total leukonychia

In this rare condition (Figure 7.1) the nail may be milky, chalky, bluish, ivory or porcelain white in colour. The opacity of the whiteness varies: when it is faintly opaque, it may be possible to see transverse streaks of leukonychia in a nail with total leukonychia. A transition to black has been observed in the distal nail plate portion in patients suffering from severe cholestatic jaundice. Accelerated nail growth may be associated with total leukonychia.

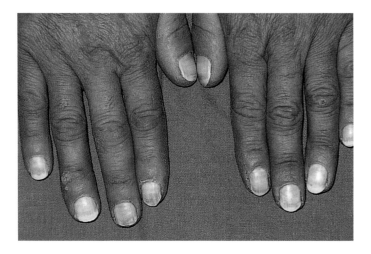

Figure 7.1
Leukonychia – hereditary type.

Subtotal leukonychia

In subtotal leukonychia there is a pink arc of about 2–4 mm in width distal to the white area. Nucleated cells in the distal area were believed to mature, lose their keratohyalin granules and then produce normal nail keratin several months after their formation. It was also suggested that parakeratotic cells are present along the whole length of the nail; these decrease in number as they approach the distal end, thus producing the normal pink colour up to the point of separation from the nail bed. There might, however, be sufficient nucleated onychocytes remaining for the nail to acquire a whitish tint after loss of contact with the nail bed. Some authorities feel that subtotal leukonychia is a phase of total leukonychia based on the occurrence of both types in different members of one family and the simultaneous occurrence in one person. In addition, either type may be found alone in some individuals at different times.

Transverse leukonychia

One or several finger nails exhibit a band, usually transverse, 1–2 mm wide and often occurring at the same site in each nail (Figures 7.2, 7.3). Transverse leukonychia is almost always due to trauma affecting the distal matrix, for example overzealous manicuring. The condition is more frequently seen in children and adolescents. There is apparently an inborn tendency to develop transverse leukonychia from minor repeated trauma.

Multiple transverse leukonychia may involve the great toes and/or the second toe nails. In these patients, whose nails are never trimmed short, the free margin is presumed to impinge

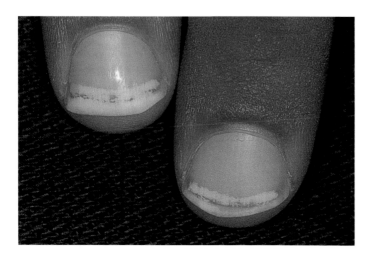

Figure 7.2
Leukonychia – transverse banded type.

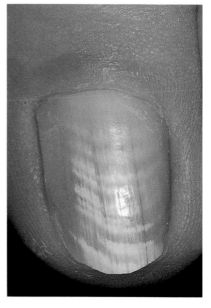

Figure 7.3
Extensive variant of the type in Figure 7.2.

on the distal part of the shoe. Cutting the affected nails short leads to complete cure.

Punctate leukonychia

Punctate leukonychia is characterized by white spots 1–3 mm in diameter occurring singly or in groups almost exclusively on finger nails. They are usually due to repeated minor trauma to the matrix. The evolution of the spots is variable; appearing generally on contact with the cuticle, they grow distally with the nail. Approximately half of them disappear as they migrate towards the free edge. This is believed to prove that parakeratotic cells are capable of maturing and losing their keratohyalin granules to produce keratin, even though they have been without a blood supply for many months. Some white spots enlarge, while others appear at a distance from the lunula, suggesting that the nail bed is participating by incorporating groups of nucleated cells into the nail. A similar process could explain the exclusively distal leukonychia which is occasionally seen. A local or general fault in keratinization is not the only cause of punctate leukonychia; infiltration of air, which is known to occur in cutaneous parakeratoses, was for a long time believed to play a part. Disturbance of the nail plate's highly organized keratin fibre system alters its transparency and makes it look white. This is evidenced by polarization microscopy, as most clinically white spots lose their birefringence.

Leukonychia variegata

Leukonychia variegata consists of white, irregular, transverse, thread-like streaks.

Isolated longitudinal leukonychia

Isolated longitudinal leukonychia is an example of localized metaplasia. It is characterized by a permanent, greyish-white longitudinal streak, 1 mm wide, below the nail plate. Histologically there is a mound of horny cells causing the white discoloration due to a lack of transparency, leading to alteration in light diffraction. Subungual filamentous tumour is the most common cause. Imbibition of blood may turn distal parts brown or even black.

Apparent leukonychia

The cause of apparent leukonychia is an alteration of the subungual tissue, either a vascular abnormality or onycholysis/nail bed hyperkeratosis.

White opacity of the nails in patients with cirrhosis is also called Terry's nails. In the majority of cases, the nails are of an opaque white colour, obscuring the lunula (Figure 7.4). This discoloration, which stops suddenly 1–2 mm from the distal edge of the nail, leaves a pink area corresponding to the onychodermal band. It lies parallel to the distal part of the nail bed and may be irregular. The condition involves all nails evenly.

A variation of Terry's nail is the Morey and Burke type in which the whitening of the nail extends to the central segment with a curved leading edge. Muehrcke's lines (Figure 7.5), which are mainly seen in hypoalbuminaemia, run parallel to the lunula and are separated from one another and from the lunula, by stripes of pink nail. They disappear when the serum albumin level returns to normal and reappear if it falls again. It is possible that hypoalbuminaemia produces oedema of the connective tissue in front of the lunula just below the epidermis of the nail bed, changing the compact arrangement of the collagen in this area to a looser texture, resembling the structure of the lunula; hence the whitish colour. The direct correlation between the presence or disappearance of the white bands and the serum

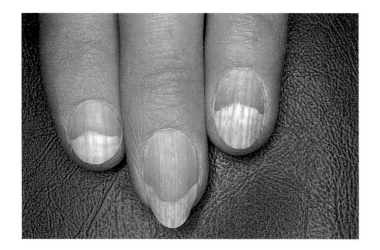

Figure 7.4
Leukonychia (apparent) due to onycholysis.

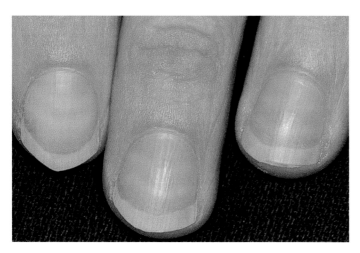

Figure 7.5
White bands due to hypoalbuminaemia (Muehrcke's lines).

albumin level appears to confirm this hypothesis. However, white finger nails preceded by multiple transverse white bands have been reported with normal serum albumin levels. Muehrcke's lines are common in patients undergoing systemic chemotherapy.

The uraemic half-and-half nail of Lindsay (Figure 7.6) consists of two parts separated more or less transversely by a well-defined line. The proximal area is dull white, resembling ground glass and obscuring the lunula; the distal area is pink, reddish or brown, and occupies between 20% and 60% of the total length of the nail (average 33%). In typical cases the diagnosis presents no difficulty, but in Terry's nail the pink, distal area may occupy up to 50% of the length of the nail; under these circumstances the two types may be confused. Half-and-half nail may display a normal proximal half, the colour of the distal part being due to an increase in the number of capillaries and thickening of their walls, or melanin granules in the nail bed. Sometimes the distinctly abnormal onychodermal band extends approximately 20–25% from the distal

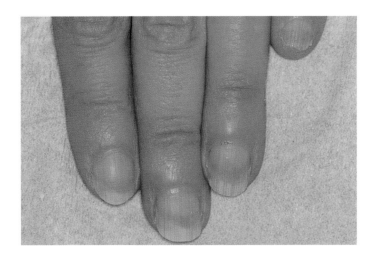

Figure 7.6
Uraemic half-and-half nail of
Lindsay.

portion of the finger nail as a distal crescent of pigmentation with pigment throughout the brown arc of the nail plate.

Nail changes similar to those reported by Terry, Lindsay and Muehrcke have been termed 'Neapolitan nails'; they are probably simply a phenomenon of old age in otherwise normal individuals.

Anaemia may produce pallor of the nail (apparent leukonychia), if the haemoglobin level falls sufficiently, similar to mucous membrane and conjunctival pallor.

Dermatoses causing leukonychia

All conditions leading to onycholysis also cause apparent leukonychia. Psoriasis may cause both true and apparent leukonychia. True leukonychia is due to matrix involvement, and apparent leukonychia to onycholysis and/or parakeratosis of the nail bed. One of the earliest signs of leprosy is apparent macrolunula, which may become total in dystrophic leprosy.

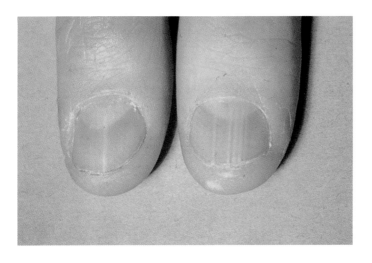

Figure 7.7
Longitudinal white lines in Hailey–Hailey disease. (Courtesy of S. Burge, UK.)

Table 7.1 Causes of leukonychia

Congenital and/or hereditary
Isolated
Acrokeratosis verruciformis (Hopf)
Associated with koilonychia (Figure 7.8)
LEOPARD syndrome (lentigines,
electrocardiographic changes, ocular
hypertelorism, pulmonary stenosis,
abnormalities of genitalia, retarded
growth, deafness)
Associated with deafness
Leukonychia totalis, multiple sebaceous
cysts, renal calculi
Darier's disease – usually linear and
longitudinal

Acquired
Pseudoleukonychia
Diffuse form of distal and lateral subungual
onychomycosis
Proximal white subungual onychomycosis,
especially in AIDS patients
Superficial white onychomycosis
Keratin granulation (superficial friability from
nail varnish)
Psoriasis
Apparent leukonychia (Figure 7.9)
Anaemia
Cancer chemotherapeutic agents
Cirrhosis (Terry's sign)
Dyshidrosis
Half-and-half nail (renal diseases) and distal
crescent pigmentation
Leprosy
Muehrcke's lines of hypoalbuminaemia

True leukonychia
Alkaline metabolic disease
Alopecia areata
Carcinoid tumours of the bronchus
Cardiac insufficiency
Cytotoxic and other drugs (emetine,
pilocarpine, sulphonamide, cortisone)
Erythema multiforme
Exfoliative dermatitis
Fasting periods (e.g. in orthodox Jews and
Muslims)
Fracture
Gout
Hodgkin's disease
Hypocalcaemia
Infectious diseases and infectious fevers
Intra-abdominal malignancies
Kidney transplant
Leprosy
Leuko-onycholysis paradentotica
Menstrual cycle
Myocardial infarction
Occupational
Pellagra
Peripheral neuropathy
Poisoning (antimony, arsenic, fluoride, lead,
thallium)
Protein deficiency
Psoriasis
Psychotic episodes (acute)
Renal failure (acute or chronic)
Shock
Sickle cell anaemia
Surgery
Sympathetic leukonychia
Trauma (single or repeated)
Tumours (benign), cysts pressing on matrix
Ulcerative colitis
Zinc deficiency

Leukonychia may also occur in other dermatoses affecting the matrix, such as alopecia areata, dyshidrosis, Darier's disease and Hailey–Hailey disease (Figure 7.7). Table 7.1 lists many of the causes and factors leading to leukonychia.

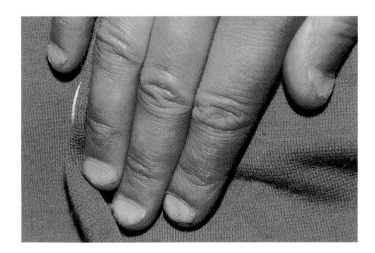

Figure 7.8
Leukokoilonychia. (Courtesy of A. Puissant, Paris.)

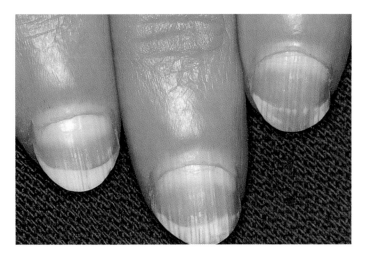

Figure 7.9
Apparent leukonychia in Raynaud's syndrome.

Pseudoleukonychia

Exogenous white stains and particularly super-ficial white onychomycosis (Jessner's leukony-chia trichophytica) cause white nails. In temperate climates the cause of superficial white onychomycosis is usually *Trichophyton mentagrophytes*, but in hot and humid climates also moulds such as *Fusarium* species may infect the surface of the nail plate. The nail is white and opaque also in proximal subungual onychomycosis and endonyx onychomycosis. Long-term application of nail varnish, layer over layer without prior removal of previous lacquer, may cause a peculiar softening and white colour of the nail surface (Table 7.1).

MELANONYCHIA (BROWN OR BLACK NAIL)

Colour change to brown or black (Figures 7.10–7.16) is potentially serious because malignant melanoma (see Chapter 5) may present in many guises; however, many less

Table 7.2 Causes of melanonychia

Black nails

Naevi (Figure 7.10)
Racial (Figure 7.11)
Drugs, e.g. doxorubicin, cyclophosphamide
Haemorrhage (Figure 7.12) (see Chapter 9)
Malignant melanoma (see Chapter 5)
Onychomycoses (*Trichophyton rubrum* var.
  nigricans, dematiaceous fungi)
Silver nitrate

Brown nails

Exogenous
  Drugs and dyes, e.g. dithranol,
    potassium permanganate (Figures
    7.13–7.16)
Endogenous
  Naevi, lentigines
  Laugier–Hunziker–Baran syndrome (see
    Chapter 5)
  Peutz–Jeghers–Touraine syndrome
  Racial (black, Asian)
  Addison's disease
  Drugs, e.g. chlorpromazine,
    tetracyclines, ketoconazole,
    sulphonamides, cytotoxics, acyclovir
  Fetal hydantoin syndrome
  Haemochromatosis
  Malnutrition
  Nail enamels and hardeners
  Pregnancy
  Thyroid disease
  Smoking, tar

Table 7.3 Causes of longitudinal melanonychia

Idiopathic

Racial

Dark skin pigmentation

Systemic

Addison's disease of the adrenal gland
Adrenalectomy for Cushing's disease
Carcinoma of the breast
Drugs
Irradiation
Malnutrition
Photochemotherapy
Pregnancy
Secondary syphilis
Vitamin B_{12} deficiency

Dermatological

Amyloid (primary)
Basal cell carcinoma
Bacterial infection
Bowen's disease
Fungal infection
Laugier–Hunziker–Baran syndrome
Lichen planus
Malignant melanoma
Peutz–Jeghers–Touraine syndrome
Porphyria cutanea tarda
Radiotherapy and radiodermatitis

Regional and local

Carpal tunnel syndrome
Repeated minor injuries
Friction
Trauma (acute or repeated)

significant abnormalities can produce brown or black discoloration (Table 7.2). Most of the causes will be self-evident at the time of presentation, either from the history or on

> **An acquired single streak of dark pigmentation is a melanoma until proved otherwise**

careful medical examination. Bearing in mind the potential risk of malignant melanoma, one should rule out the other conditions that may present with this sign (Table 7.3). When no specific cause is found, the following features

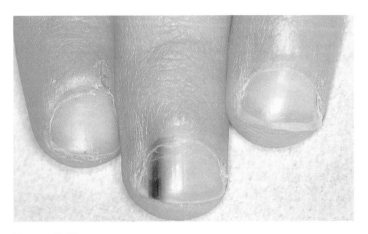

Figure 7.10
Longitudinal melanonychia – congenital naevus.

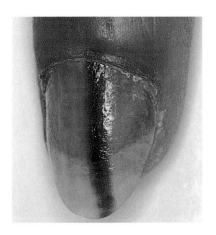

Figure 7.11
Aquired longitudinal melanonychia.

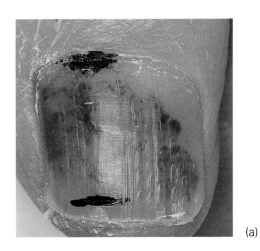

(a)

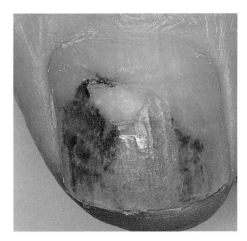

(b)

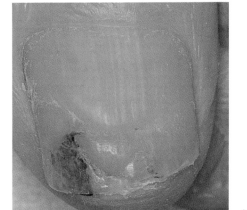

(c)

Figure 7.12
(a, b, c) Subungual haematoma
showing slow resolution.

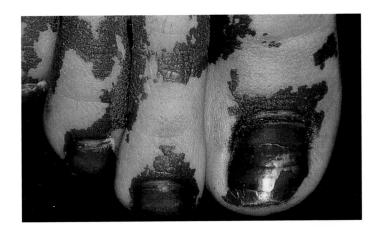

Figure 7.13
Fuchsin nail staining – Castellani's paint.

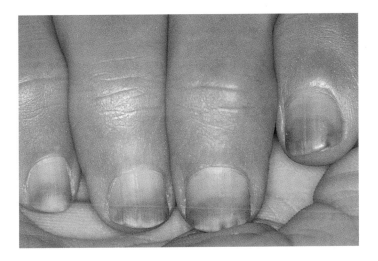

Figure 7.14
Brown staining due to henna.

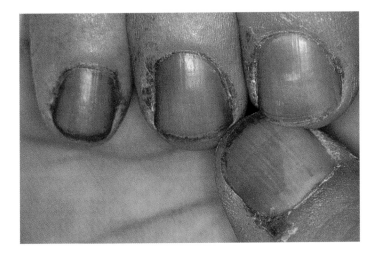

Figure 7.15
Silver nitrate staining.

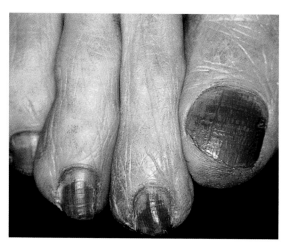

Figure 7.16
Brown staining due to potassium permanganate.

should be considered indicative of possible malignant melanoma:

- only one digit affected
- periungual spread of the pigmentation
- darkening of an established band
- progressive widening of the linear streak with blurring of its border
- age over 50 years.

Linear pigmentation not reaching the free edge of the nail is unlikely to be due to a melanocytic focus in the matrix.

The following conditions should also be excluded:

- associated non-melanoma periungual pigmentation (pseudo-Hutchinson's sign)
- single longitudinal melanonychia due to metastases of distant malignant melanoma
- non-migratory haematoma or foreign body.

The dangers of misdiagnosis are:

1 Proper treatment of subungual melanoma may be delayed, leading to tumour spread and even death.

Table 7.4 Some causes of discoloration

Yellow
Yellow nail syndrome (Figure 7.18)
Nail enamel and hardeners
AIDS
Carotene
Dermatophyte onychomycosis (see Chapter 8)
Drugs, e.g. tetracycline (fluorescent lunula), penicillamine, clioquinole (topical), mepacrine (nail bed)
Jaundice

Blue to grey
Antimalarials (Figure 7.19)
Argyria
Bleomycin
Congenital pernicious anaemia
Minocycline
Phenolphthalein
Phenothiazines
Wilson's disease

Green
Aspergillus
Bullous disorders
Jaundice
'Old' haematoma (green-yellow)
Pseudomonas aeruginosa (Figure 7.20)

Red/purple
Angioma
Cirsoid aneurysm tumour
Glomus tumour (see Figures 3.8, 5.25)
Congestive cardiac failure (lunula) (Figure 7.21)
Enchodroma
Heparin (transverse)
Lichen planus
Linear red line
    Darier's disease
    Benign tumours or cysts near proximal matrix
Lupus erythematosus
Porphyria (with fluorescent light)
Rheumatoid arthritis
Warfarin

2 Treatment for subungual melanoma may lead to overtreatment of a benign lesion and thus to unnecessary surgery. Excision biopsy is therefore crucial.

Potassium permanganate was often used in the past as a disinfectant for hand and foot baths. Brown staining of the skin and nails was regularly observed. Whereas the stained horny layer soon desquamated, the nails remained dirty brown owing to deposition of manganium dioxide on the nail surface. This can be easily removed by reducing manganium dioxide with ascorbic acid: a small gauze pad is moistened with ascorbic acid solution and used to vigorously wipe the nail surface.

Silver nitrate stains the nail jet-black. The stained nail grows out with a contour parallel to the border of the proximal nail fold. Histopathology has shown black silver nitrate globules penetrating approximately the superficial third of the nail plate; this is the reason that it cannot be easily removed with ammonium compounds.

OTHER DISCOLORATIONS

The varieties of colour change that may occur in the nail apparatus (other than white and brown-black) are listed in Table 7.4, and some examples are shown in Figures 7.17–7.21. Many are due to obvious cosmetic procedures, topical or oral drugs, application of antiseptics (Figure 7.17) or common diseases. None of them is of any particular significance, their presence sometimes aiding in the diagnosis of disease or pointing towards overdose of drugs.

Greenish-black discoloration is typical of *Pseudomonas aeruginosa* infection (Figure 7.20). It often starts at one side of a finger nail, growing out from under the proximal nail fold. A slight thickening of the latter and breaks in the cuticle may accompany the condition. Treatment is difficult since part of the infection is hidden and not amenable to topical treatment. Even though the condition is harmless for the patient it may cause life-threatening infections in immunocompromised persons. Nurses with this *Pseudomonas* infection should not work in operation room facilities or with immunocompromised patients.

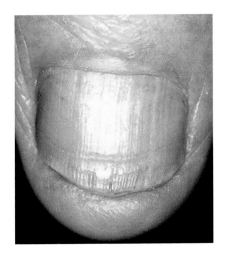

Figure 7.17
Stain due to copper in antiseptic solution.

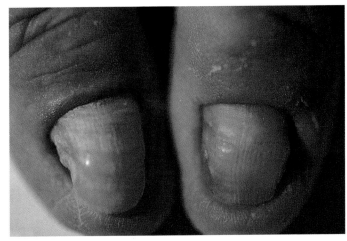

Figure 7.18
Yellow nail syndrome.

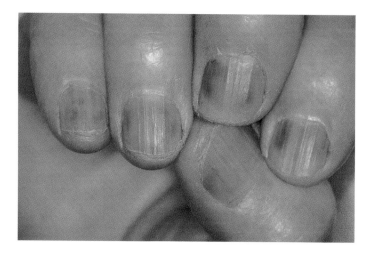

Figure 7.19
Nail discoloration due to systemic antimalarial treatment.

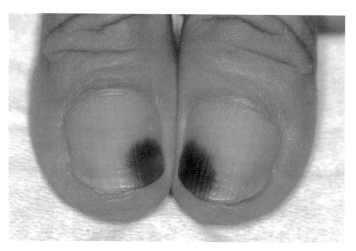

Figure 7.20
Pseudomonas colonization of onycholysis leaving nail plate pyocyanin stain.

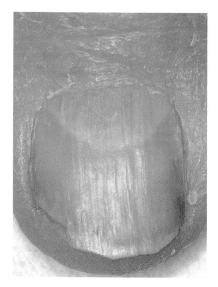

Figure 7.21
Red lunulae – occasionally seen in heart failure and alopecia areata.

Red lunulae may be seen in particularly severe, acute nail involvement in erythema multiforme, Stevens–Johnson syndrome, Lyell's syndrome, generalized psoriasis, alopecia areata, systemic lupus erythematosus, dermatomyositis and rheumatoid arthritis, among other conditions (Figure 7.21).

FURTHER READING

Melanonychia

Baran R, Haneke E (1984) Diagnostik und Therapie der streifenformigen Nagelpigmentierung, *Hautarzt* **35**: 359–365.

Baran R, Kechijian P (1989) Longitudinal melanonychia (melanonychia striata): diagnosis and management, *J Am Acad Dermatol* **21**: 1165–1175.

Other discolorations

Daniel CR (1985) Nail pigmentation abnormalities, *Dermatol Clin* **3**: 431–443.

8 Onychomycosis and its treatment

Antonella Tosti, Robert Baran, Rodney PR Dawber, Eckart Haneke

Types of onychomycosis • Diagnosis • Treatment • Candida onychomycosis • Further reading

Fungi may invade the nails in four different ways, leading to four separate types of onychomycosis with specific clinical features, prognosis and response to treatment. The type of nail invasion depends on the fungus responsible and the host susceptibility. Invasion occurs:

1   Via the distal subungual area and the lateral nail groove, leading to distal lateral subungual onychomycosis (Figure 8.1).

2   Via the undersurface of the proximal nail fold leading to proximal subungual onychomycosis (see Figure 8.10).

3   Via the dorsal surface of the nail plate, producing superficial onychomycosis (see Figure 8.16).

4   Via the nail plate free margin, producing endonyx onychomycosis (see Figure 8.21).

Table 8.1 Causes of onychomycosis

Type of organism	Prevalence (%)
Dermatophytes	83
Non-dermatophytic moulds	15 (approx.)
Yeasts	< 1

TYPES OF ONYCHOMYCOSIS

Distal lateral subungual onychomycosis

Distal lateral subungual onychomycosis (DLSO) is the most common type of onychomycosis (Figures 8.3, 8.4, 8.5, 8.7–8.9). Responsible

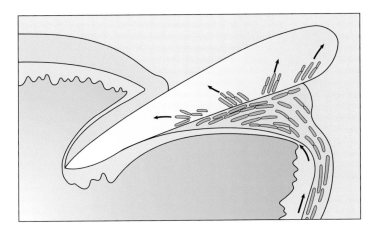

Figure 8.1
Nail invasion in distal lateral subungual onychomycosis.

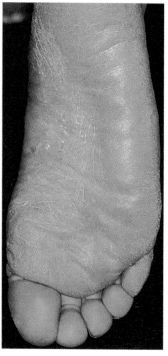

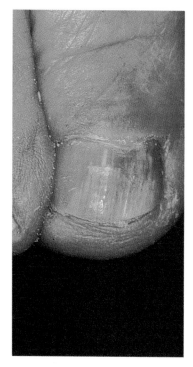

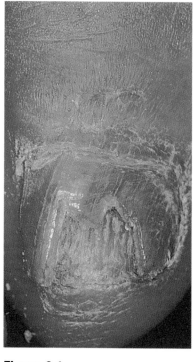

Figure 8.2
Plantar scaling due to
Trichophyton rubrum
infection in a patient with
DLSO.

Figure 8.3
Nail bed hyperkeratosis and
onycholysis of the great toe
in DLSO.

Figure 8.4
The hyperkeratotic nail bed in
DLSO is evident after clipping of
the detached nail plate.

Figure 8.5
Distal lateral subungual
onychomycosis of several fingers.

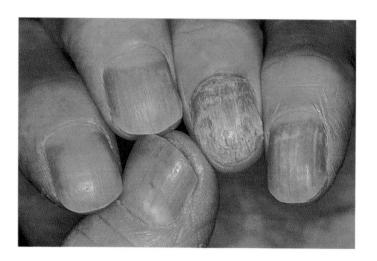

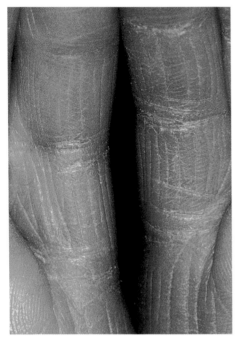

Figure 8.6
Palmar involvement in the patient
shown in Figure 8.5.

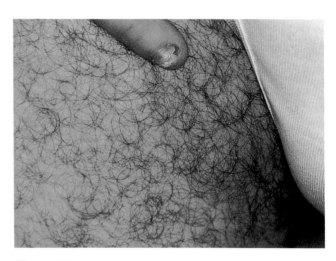

Figure 8.7
Tinea cruris in a patient affected by DLSO of several
finger nails due to *Trichophyton rubrum*.

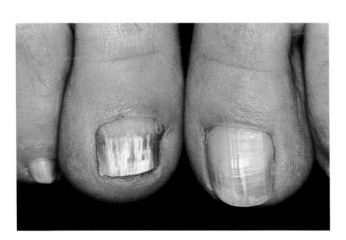

Figure 8.8
Distal lateral subungual onychomycosis due to
Fusarium solanii.

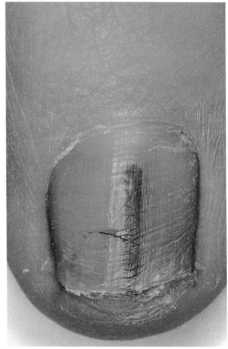

Figure 8.9
Fungal melanonychia due to
Trichophyton rubrum.

fungi (Table 8.1) include dermatophytes (most frequently *Trichophyton rubrum*), moulds (*Scytalidium* spp., *Scopulariopsis* spp., *Fusarium* spp., *Acremonium* spp., *Onychocola canadensis*) and yeasts (*Candida* spp.). The skin of the palms and soles is frequently involved, especially in dermatophytic infections with plantar scaling (Figure 8.2). Tinea cruris is common in patients with onychomycosis due to *T. rubrum* and *Epidermophyton floccosum* (see Figure 8.7).

Toe nails are most frequently affected (Figure 8.3). Finger nail infection is usually associated with toe nail infection, often presenting as the 'one hand, two feet' syndrome. Clinically the nail shows distal subungual hyperkeratosis and onycholysis; the onycholytic area appears yellow–white. Proximal spreading frequently occurs along longitudinal streaks. In some cases the nail plate is partially absent, the detached nail having been clipped by the patient (Figure 8.4).

Yellow streaks along the lateral margin of the nail and/or the presence of yellow onycholytic areas in the central portion of the nail (dermatophytoma) are associated with poor response to systemic antifungal medication. A poor prognosis is also reported for onychomycosis due to some moulds such as *Scytalidium*, *Scopulariopsis* and *Fusarium*, or for onychomycosis due to *T. rubrum* var. *melanoides*. The latter dermatophyte produces black pigmentation of the nail due to direct production of melanin-related pigment by the fungus (Figure 8.9).

Proximal subungual onychomycosis

Fungi reach the nail matrix keratogenous zone through the proximal nail fold horny layer (Figure 8.10) and are typically located in the ventral nail (Figures 8.11–8.15). Proximal subungual onychomycosis (PSO) is most frequently caused by moulds (*Scopulariopsis brevicaulis*, *Fusarium* spp. and *Aspergillus* spp.). It may also be caused

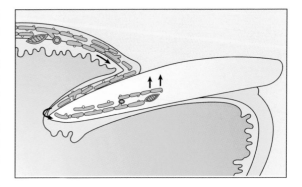

Figure 8.10
Nail invasion in proximal subungual onychomycosis.

by *Trichophyton rubrum* in people infected with human immunodeficiency virus (HIV). Finger nail invasion is rare. Proximal subungual onychomycosis presents as an area of leukonychia in the proximal portion of the nail plate; the leukonychia is due to the presence of fungal elements in the ventral portion of the proximal nail plate. The nail plate surface is normal. When PSO is caused by moulds, the periungual tissues are frequently inflamed and the condition may closely resemble a bacterial infection. A purulent discharge may be present, especially in *Aspergillus* infection. When PSO affects finger nails or the thin nails of children, fungal invasion may spread to the dorsal nail layers, resulting in opacity and fragility of the superficial nail plate. This has been frequently reported under the diagnosis of 'white superficial onychomycosis'.

Superficial onychomycosis

Superficial onychomycosis (Figures 8.16–8.20) only affects toe nails. Most commonly the responsible fungus is *Trichophyton Mentagrophytes* var. *interdigitale*, but moulds (*Fusarium*, *Acremonium* and *Aspergillus*) can also be responsible (Table 8.2). The nail shows small, white opaque patches that can be easily

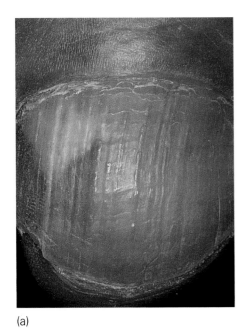

(a)

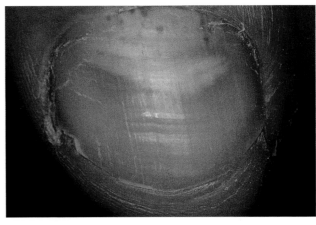

(b)

Figure 8.11
(a, b) Proximal subungual onychomycosis: the proximal nail shows an area of leukonychia. The nail surface is normal.

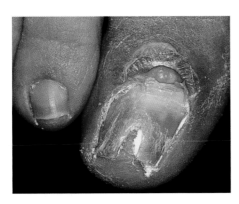

Figure 8.12
Proximal subungual onychomycosis due to *Aspergillus flavus* – note periungual inflammation with purulent discharge.

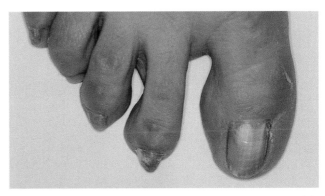

(a)

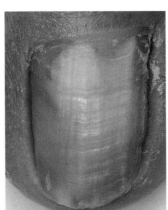

(b)

Figure 8.13
(a, b) Proximal subungual onychomycosis with periungual inflammation due to *Scopulariopsis brevicaulis*.

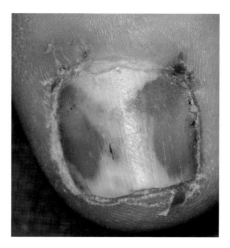

Figure 8.14
Fingernail PSO due to *Fusarium* sp.
– note leukonychia and periungual
inflammation.

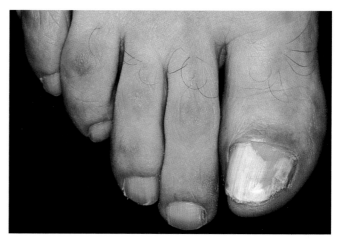

Figure 8.15
Proximal subungual onychomycosis due to *Fusarium* sp.
– note erythema of the proximal nail fold.

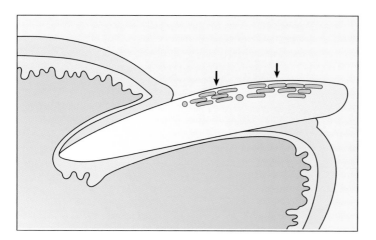

Figure 8.16
Nail invasion in white superficial onychomycosis.

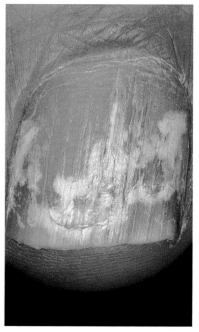

Figure 8.17
The nail plate surface in WSO
presents numerous white,
opaque and friable spots.

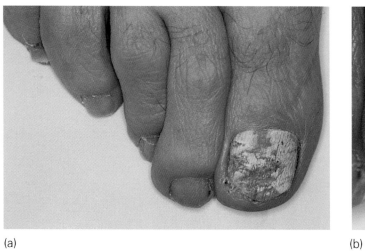

(a)

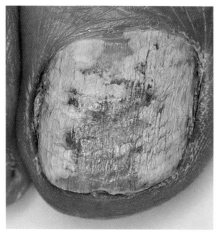

(b)

Figure 8.18
(a, b) White superficial onychomycosis due to *Aspergillus candidus*.

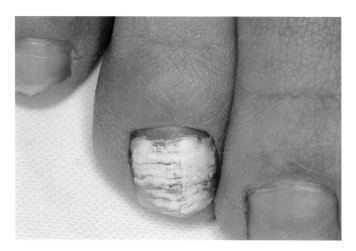

Figure 8.19
White superficial onychomycosis due to *Fusarium* sp.

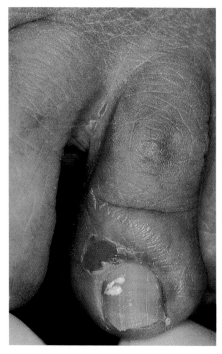

Figure 8.20
Tinea pedis interdigitalis in a patient with WSO.

scraped off (white superficial onychomycosis, WSO). Tinea pedis interdigitalis is frequently associated. Children presenting with WSO may have *Candida* infection.

Trichophyton rubrum var. *melanoides* and *Scytalydium dimidiatum* can be responsible for a rare variety of superficial onychomycosis, black superficial onychomycosis, in which the patches are black.

Endonyx onychomycosis

Endonyx onychomycosis (Figures 8.21, 8.22) is a rare type of onychomycosis caused by

Trichophyton soudanense and *T. violaceum*. Plantar infection may be associated (Figure 8.23). The nail is diffusely opaque and white in the absence of onycholysis and subungual hyperkeratosis.

Total dystrophic onychomycosis

Total dystrophic onychomycosis (TDO) may rarely occur as a primary condition or, most commonly, represent the secondary evolution of untreated DLSO or PSO. Primary TDO is usually due to *Candida* and typically affects immunocompromised people, such as

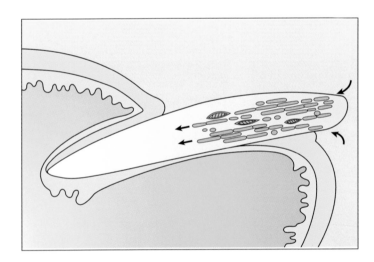

Figure 8.21
Schematic drawing of nail invasion in endonyx onychomycosis.

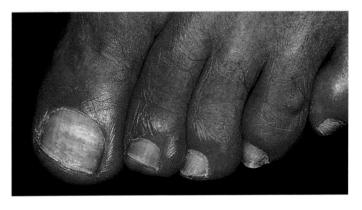

Figure 8.22
Milky-white discoloration of the nail plate in endonyx onychomycosis in the absence of subungual hyperkeratosis and onycholysis.

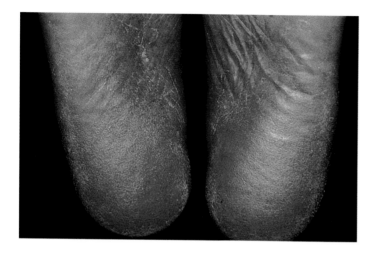

Figure 8.23
Plantar infection due to *Trichophyton soudanense* in the patient seen in Figure 8.22.

patients with chronic mucocutaneous candidiasis or HIV infection. The nail is diffusely thickened and crumbled, and the periungual tissues are inflamed with pseudoclubbing.

DIAGNOSIS

Diagnosis of dermatophyte nail invasion can be established by the isolation and identification of the fungi from the affected nail, provided that no local or systemic antifungal treatment has been used recently by the patient. The site from which diagnostic specimens should be taken depends on the type of onychomycosis:

- In DLSO subungual debris should be collected from the nail bed after clipping off the overlying onycholytic nail plate (Figure 8.24). It is important to obtain material from the most proximal portion of the affected nail bed.
- In PSO fungi are restricted to the ventral nail plate. When the affected area is far from the distal edge of the nail, collection of the specimens requires punch biopsy of the nail plate.

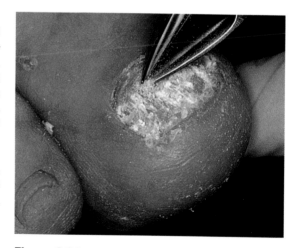

Figure 8.24
Collection of specimens in DSO. Subungual debris should be collected in the most proximal portion of the affected nail bed after clipping of the onycholytic nail plate.

> **Finger nail fungal infection is rare in the absence of toe nail involvement or tinea pedis**

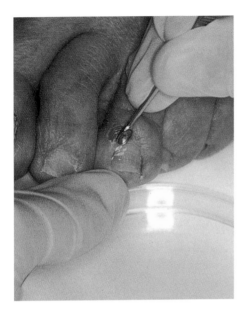

Figure 8.25
Collection of specimens in WSO. Nail debris
can be obtained by scraping the areas of
leukonychia on the superficial nail plate.

• In WSO the material can easily be obtained
  by scraping the areas of leukonychia or
  melanonychia from the superficial nail plate
  (Figure 8.25).

• In endonyx onychomycosis nail clippings
  contain numerous fungal elements and can
  be used directly for culture.

Direct microscopic examination of the specimens can be performed using potassium
hydroxide preparations. Nail debris is placed on
a glass slide and a drop of a 40% KOH solution
with ink (3 ml of KOH solution mixed with 1
cartridge of ink) added. After applying a cover-
slip, the slide is placed in a moist chamber for
2 hours to permit clearing of the keratin; it is
then viewed under a microscope (Figures
8.26–8.28). A formulation of KOH and
dimethylsulphoxide (DMSO) provides faster
clearing of the specimen. Samples are cultured
in Sabouraud's medium with 0.05% chloramphenicol with or without 0.4% cycloheximide,
incubated at 26–28°C for 2–3 weeks. Gross
colony morphology and microscopic examination of the mycelia stained with lactophenol
cotton blue permit the identification of the
causative fungus (Figures 8.29–8.31).
  The failure rate for nail culture is high
(20–30%) since fungi may be scarcely visible
and fail to grow. When the clinical picture and
direct examination are indicative of onychomycosis it is mandatory to repeat the culture.
Examination of material taken from associated

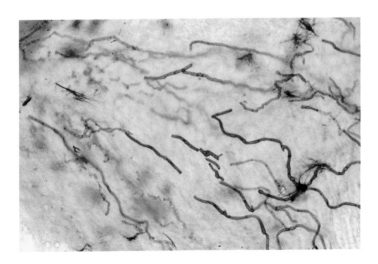

Figure 8.26
Nail preparation in 40% KOH and
ink showing dermatophyte
filaments.

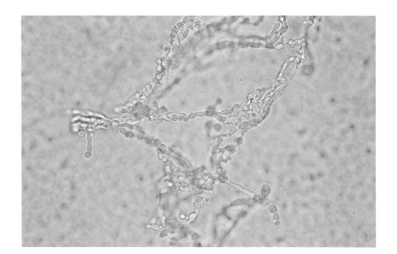

Figure 8.27
Scopulariopsis brevicaulis onychomycosis: KOH preparation showing the lemon-shaped conidia.

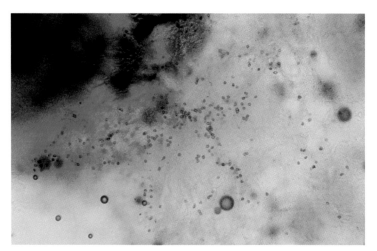

Figure 8.28
Onychomycosis due to *Aspergillus niger.* KOH preparation showing several black conidial heads visible within the nail plate.

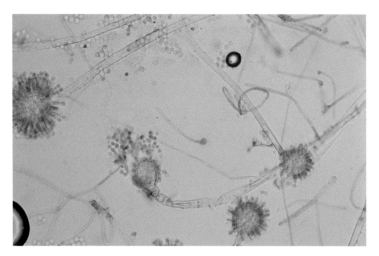

Figure 8.29
Aspergillus niger in culture.

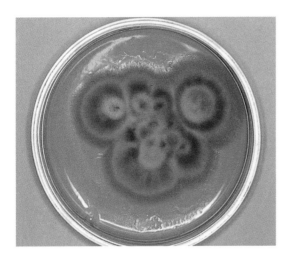

Figure 8.30
Culture of *Trichophyton rubrum* on Sabouraud's medium after 20 days' incubation at 26°C.

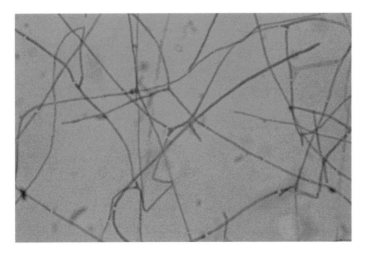

Figure 8.31
Microscopic examination of a culture of *Trichophyton soudanense* showing septate hyphae with reflexive branching and chains of arthrospores.

skin lesions is advisable since these usually give profuse dermatophyte growth. Diagnosis of onychomycosis due to moulds requires a strict correlation between clinical picture and mycological results. Isolation of a mould from culture is not a sufficient criterion to make the

diagnosis, since moulds may be contaminants or secondary colonizers of the nail as well as laboratory contaminants.

Differential diagnosis

Differentiating between onychomycosis and psoriasis can be difficult since subungual hyperkeratosis, onycholysis, splinter haemorrhages and diffuse nail 'crumbling' are clinical signs of both conditions. Moreover, dermatophytes or

---

Onychomycosis may be secondary to other factors – important to consider if treatment fails

other fungi can occasionally colonize psoriatic nails, especially when the nail plate is grossly deformed. Therefore, positive culture does not exclude the diagnosis of psoriasis.

TREATMENT

Except for superficial onychomycosis, which can be treated with any topical antifungal agent after scraping of the affected areas, treatment of dermatophyte onychomycosis usually requires systemic antifungal therapy. However, when only the distal nail is affected and the patient's general condition makes systemic treatment questionable, topical therapy using the transungual drug delivery system (TUDDS) can be tried, using daily 8% ciclopirox or weekly 5% amorolfine nail lacquer. Therapy should be continued for at least 6 months in finger nail onychomycosis and 12 months in toe nail infection: 8% ciclopirox once daily, 5% amorolfine nail lacquer once or twice weekly. A combination of bifonazole 1% in a 40% urea ointment is a possible alternative.

Formerly oral treatment of onychomycosis consisted of two antifungal drugs: griseofulvin and ketoconazole, the latter being rarely used in recent years because of its hepatotoxicity. Treatment of onychomycosis with griseofulvin, however, requires long-term administration of the drug (6 months for finger nails, up to 18 months for toe nails), and high drug dosages (up to 2 g per day). Toe nail infection often fails to respond and recurrence is common. Three new systemic antimycotic agents have now been introduced: fluconazole, itraconazole and terbinafine. All these drugs have been shown to reach the distal nail soon after therapy is started and to persist in the nail plate for long periods (2–6 months) after the end of treatment. The persistence of high drug levels in the nail following treatment allows for shorter treatment periods with fewer relapses and side-effects. Partial nail avulsion and concomitant treatment with a topical antifungal agent further reduce relapses and shorten the duration of treatment. Onychomycosis of the toe nails is more difficult to cure and recurs more frequently than onychomycosis of the finger nails.

Fluconazole and itraconazole are triazole derivatives with a broad spectrum of fungistatic activity. Itraconazole is effective at dosages of 200 mg per day for 2–4 months. This agent has been shown to be effective even when given as intermittent therapy (400 mg daily for 1 week every month for 3–6 months). Terbinafine is an allylamine derivative with primary fungicidal properties against dermatophytes. This drug is probably more effective and safer than other antimycotics for long-term treatment of onychomycosis due to dermatophytes. Recommended dosage is 250 mg per day for 2 months (finger nails) to 4 months (toe nails). Preliminary studies show that terbinafine may also be effective at the dosage of 500 mg daily for 1 week a month (intermittent therapy).

When onychomycosis is cured it is advisable to continue application of a topical conventional antifungal agent on the previously affected nails, soles and toe webs to reduce the chance of relapse, unless the new transungual antifungal delivery systems (5% amorolfine and 8% ciclopirox) are used in a preventive manner.

CANDIDA ONYCHOMYCOSIS

Candida albicans can frequently be isolated from the subungual area of onycholytic nails as well as from the proximal nail fold of chronic paronychia. In both these conditions, however, *Candida* colonization is only a secondary

> ***Candida* invasion of the nail is always a secondary phenomenon, due to local or systemic factors**

Table 8.2 Routes of nail invasion by non-dermatophytic moulds

	Distal	Proximal	Superficial
Scopulariopsis brevicaulis	+	+	−
Fusarium spp.	+	+	+
Acremonium spp.	+	−	+
Aspergillus spp.	+	+	+
Scytalydium spp.	+	+	+
Onychocola canadensis	+	−	−
Alternaria spp.	+	−	−

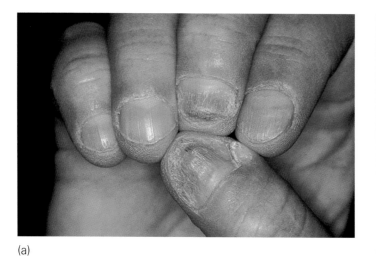

(a)

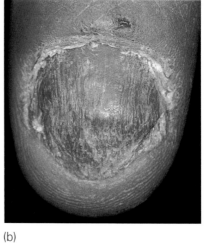

(b)

Figure 8.32
(a, b) *Candida* onychomycosis in a patient with HIV infection.

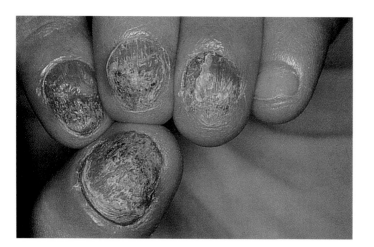

Figure 8.33
Candida onychomycosis in a child with chronic mucocutaneous candidiasis.

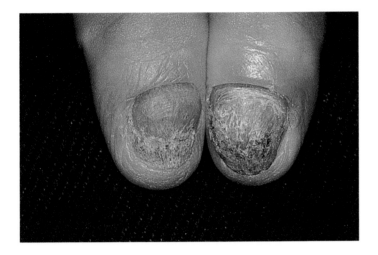

Figure 8.34
Chronic mucocutaneous candidiasis: the affected digits have a bulbous appearance with erythema and swelling of the proximal and lateral nail folds. The nail bed is hyperkeratotic and the nail plate is thickened and highly dystrophic due to diffuse crumbling. Complete destruction of the nail plate is commonly observed.

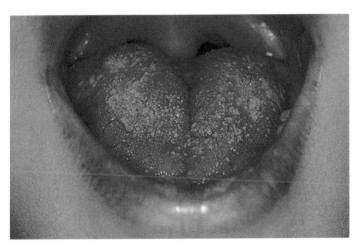

Figure 8.35
Oral candidiasis in the patient seen in Figure 8.33.

phenomenon since topical or systemic antimycotics do not cure the nail abnormalities. Nail invasion by *Candida albicans* usually indicates an underlying immunological defect (Figure 8.32) and is almost exclusively seen in chronic mucocutaneous candidiasis; in the latter, *Candida albicans* invasion of the nail plate is associated with an inflammatory reaction of the proximal nail fold, nail matrix, nail bed and hyponychium (Figure 8.33). The affected digits have a bulbous appearence with erythema and swelling of the proximal and lateral nail folds. The nail bed is hyperkeratotic and the nail plate is thickened and highly dystrophic owing to diffuse 'crumbling'. Complete destruction of the nail plate is commonly observed (Figure 8.34). Oral candidiasis is present in almost all patients (Figure 8.35).

Diagnosis

The diagnosis of candida nail invasion is made by culturing nail scrapings in Sabouraud's medium at 37°C. Isolated *Candida* strains should be tested for sensitivity to imidazoles.

Treatment

Nail lesions of chronic mucocutaneous candidiasis require systemic treatment. Ketoconazole (400 mg daily) and itraconazole (200 mg daily) are both effective, the latter having a safer side-effect profile.

FURTHER READING

Baran R, Dawber RPR (1994) *Diseases of The Nails and Their Management*, 2nd edn (Oxford, Blackwell Scientific).

Baran R, Hay RJ, Tosti A *et al* (1998) New classification of onychomycosis, *Br J Dermatol* **119**: 567–571.

Baran R, Hay R, Haneke E *et al* (1999) *Onychomycosis. The Current Approach to Diagnosis and Therapy* (London, Martin Dunitz).

Haneke E (1991) Fungal infection of the nail, *Semin Dermatol* **10**: 41–53.

Tosti A, Piraccini BM, Lorenzi S (2000) Onychomycosis caused by non-dermatophytic moulds: chemical features and response to treatment of 59 cases, *J Am Acad Dermatol* **42**: 217–224.

Zaias N (1985) Onychomycosis, *Dermatol Clin* **3**: 445–460.

9 Traumatic disorders of the nail

Rodney PR Dawber and Ivan Bristow

**Major trauma • Repeated microtrauma of the nail apparatus •
The painful nail • Further reading**

This chapter looks at three distinct aspects of trauma, under the headings:

1 Major trauma (involving any digit).
2 Repeated microtrauma.
3 The painful nail.

MAJOR TRAUMA

This section considers major trauma, single overwhelming injury, necessitating only minor 'office' surgery. Complex laceration and most of the traumatic abnormalities are beyond the intended scope of this book. Damage from acute trauma may have immediate and/or delayed effects.

Haematoma

Acute subungual haematoma is usually obvious (Figures 9.1–9.3), occurring shortly after painful trauma, for example a car door slammed on fingers or a heavy object dropped on a toe nail. The blood that accumulates under the nail plate intensifies the pain, which is severe. This prevents delay in the regrowth of the nail and secondary onychodystrophy resulting from pressure on the matrix caused by the accumulated blood. The technique used to drain the blood depends on the size of the haematoma.

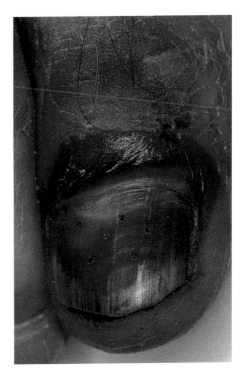

Figure 9.1
Severe traumatic haematoma.

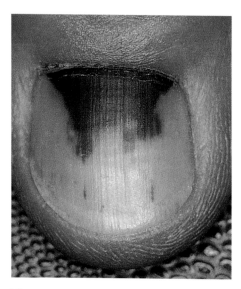

Figure 9.2
Matrix haematoma migrating distally into the nail bed.

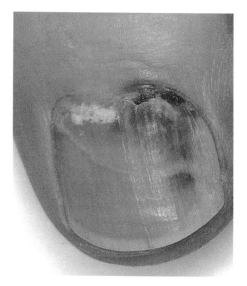

Figure 9.3
Haematoma causing partial onychomadesis.

Partial haematoma

Splinter haemorrhages are produced by the disruption of small vessels of the dermal ridges of the nail bed. They are more common in males than in females and in the first three fingers of each hand. With increased trauma, more dermal ridges are involved, resulting in ecchymoses. Subungual haematoma usually appears shortly after trauma, but if the injury occurs below the proximal nail fold, the haemorrhage may not be visible for 2–3 days. Haemorrhage in the matrix is incorporated into the nail plate; bleeding distal to the lunula remains subungual.

Total haematoma

Haematoma involving more than 25% of the visible nail is a warning sign of severe nail bed injury and possible underlying phalangeal fracture; an X-ray is therefore mandatory.

Potential development of osteterminalisitis (infection under the nail) is a hazard, as such infection can spread quickly, affecting the underlying nail structures.

Nail shedding

Nail shedding may occur acutely either by direct force or following subungual haematoma; it may also appear some months after the event.

Acute paronychia

Acute paronychia may result from a penetrating thorn or splinter into the nail fold. Infection is usually painful and due to *Staphylococcus aureus*. Systemic antibiotic therapy is indicated at an early stage. If response does not occur within 2 days, then removal of the proximal portion of the nail plate is indicated.

Pyogenic granuloma

Pyogenic granuloma (Figure 9.4) is a benign haemangioma which typically follows skin injury. It may develop in the nail bed after a penetrating wound of the nail plate. Tenderness and a tendency to bleed easily are characteristic features. Pyogenic granuloma may be removed by excision at its base, followed by the use of aluminium chloride solution as a haemostat. Histological examination is essential to rule out amelanotic melanoma.

Delayed effects of major trauma

These are numerous (Figures 9.5–9.8). Trauma-induced Beau's line accompanied by pyogenic granuloma of the proximal nail folds of the affected fingers from trauma on the palm and the arm has been reported. Delayed

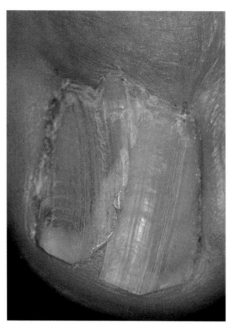

Figure 9.5
Post-traumatic fissures.

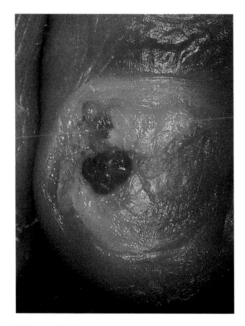

Figure 9.4
Pyogenic granuloma.

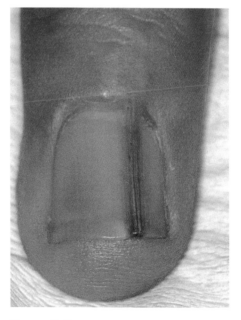

Figure 9.6
Post-traumatic nail ridge.

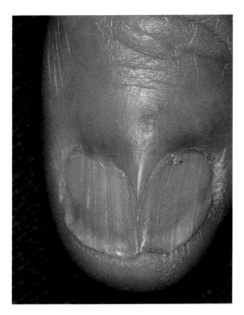

Figure 9.7
Post-traumatic nail dystrophy – pterygium scar.

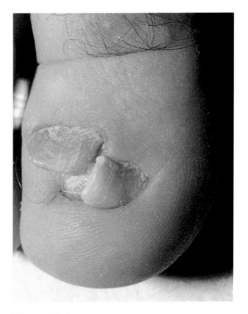

Figure 9.8
Traumatic matrix distortion and nail plate
dystrophy – ectopic nail.

Figure 9.9
'Tented' nail over a bony
exostosis.

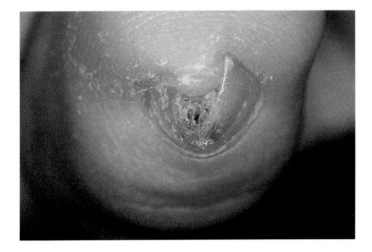

effects of major trauma include permanent
damage of the nail matrix, sometimes with
unequal growth of different sections of the nail
plate. Damage to the matrix may result in a
split extending along the entire length of the
nail, or a longitudinal prominent ridge, and may
even result in ectopic nail due to the altered
position of the matrix following the trauma.
Trauma to the proximal nail fold may be
responsible for the formation of pterygium.

Longitudinal melanonychia following acute trauma is rare in white individuals. Hook nail is observed when the nail bed is shortened after distal section of the bony phalanx. Any traumatic force to the distal phalanx can result in bony changes affecting the future nail structure. An example of this is the subungual exostosis which often leads to onychocryptosis with a 'tented' hallux nail whose lateral and medial edges impinge on their corresponding nail grooves (Figure 9.9). Significant injury was thought to be associated with the development of some cases of subungual melanoma; this is still debatable.

REPEATED MICROTRAUMA OF THE NAIL APPARATUS

Chronic trauma implies repeated minor injury often unnoticed by the patient. A history of nail trauma as a cause of onychodystrophy can therefore be more difficult to elicit. Repeated microtrauma to the toe nail is a frequent cause of nail disorders, and when assessing them it is important to take a full view of the whole foot and lower limb. All too often, practitioners treat the foot and nail as static anatomical structures when common problems arise as a result of their dynamic functions. It is only when this is taken into account that the distinct differences between finger and toe nails becomes apparent. Microtrauma to the toe nail frequently arises as a result of:

- foot function
- foot and digit shape
- footwear
- other factors.

When presented with a toe nail problem, assessment of the foot and toes should always include the weight bearing and walking by the patient to fully appreciate foot and toe position.

Foot function

In simple terms the human foot has evolved to carry out a specific function – to assist smooth and efficient locomotion. In undertaking this task the foot has developed the ability to alter its structure within a single footstep. To understand this we must briefly look at the normal gait cycle (Figure 9.10). During normal walking, the first stage (heel strike) begins when the heel comes into contact with the ground. To permit shock absorption the foot must become a flexible unit. It does this by pronation (a triplanar movement occurring mainly at the subtalar and midtarsal joints). This may be recognized by eversion of the calcaneum, lowering of the arch and slight elongation of the foot. Subtalar joint pronation unlocks the midtarsal joint so that effectively the foot is flexible to accommodate ground reaction at heel strike. The pronation occurs until the whole foot is flat to the floor (midstance or full foot). In order for this foot to take the full body weight as the opposite foot leaves the ground, it must now become a rigid unit. Once the opposite limb has passed the plantigrade foot, and undergoes heel strike, the foot begins propulsion. The heel lifts, so that body weight is shifted onto the forefoot and the toes. In order to stabilize the foot and balance the whole body forward, the foot becomes supinated (this is a movement involving the subtalar and midtarsal joints whereby the calcaneum inverts, the arch is raised and the foot is effectively shortened). This movement effectively locks the foot into rigidity, allowing a stable platform for propulsion.

Many abnormal foot functions can upset this sequence of supination–pronation–resupination. In terms of toe nail pathology, these predominantly occur around the propulsive phase of the gait cycle. If for any reason the foot has been unable to supinate to an adequate degree, there may not be sufficient rigidity and so propulsion occurs on a flexible foot. So major forces may be dissipated through the forefoot. When repeated many hundreds of times a day, this can have adverse

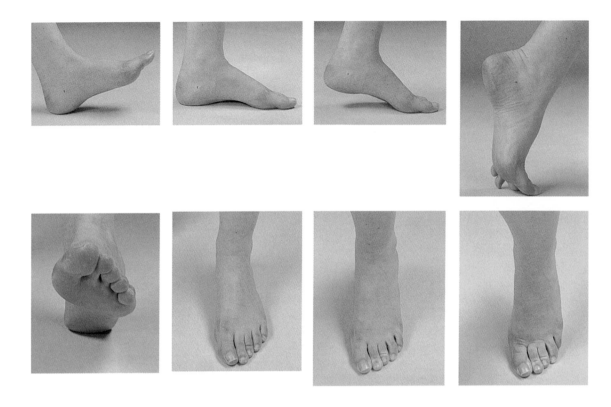

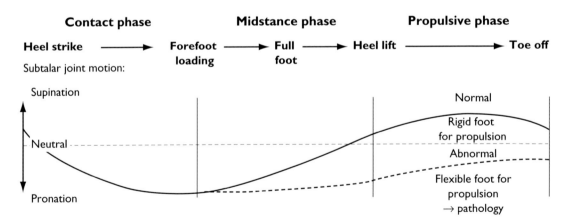

Figure 9.10
The positions of the foot during the normal gait cycle.

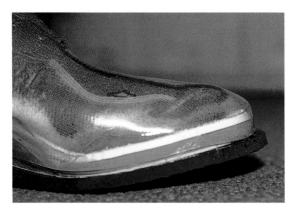

Figure 9.11
Transparent shoe demonstrating effect of shallow toe box: the hallux is compressed into the upper of the shoe.

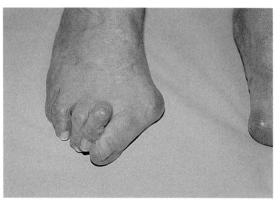

Figure 9.12
Hallux valgus.

effects on the digital area, especially when interacting with footwear. If a foot is excessively pronating on propulsion, the foot will elongate (as part of pronation) so the distal area will be subject to trauma if the footwear depth is inadequate in length (Figure 9.11). Control of excess pronation may be obtained by way of prescribed orthoses in footwear.

Foot and digit shape

Within any population there is a great variation in foot shape and it is likely that this shape will change with the effects of ageing and disease. The hallux is the digit most commonly affected by traumatic disorders. Hallux valgus (Figure 9.12) is a common orthopaedic disorder which may lead to nail problems. Gradual medial rotation of the digit occurs at the same time the hallux deviates laterally. This deformity may cause pronounced changes in the nail apparatus such as hyperkeratotic build-up along the edge of the tibial nail sulcus (Figure 9.13) and ingrowing toe nail. Lateral deviation of the hallux may lead to displacement of the second toe, which subsequently may be displaced dorsally. Counter pressure from the

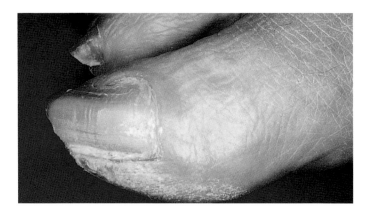

Figure 9.13
Nail dystrophy due to hallux valgus. (Courtesy of B. Schubert.)

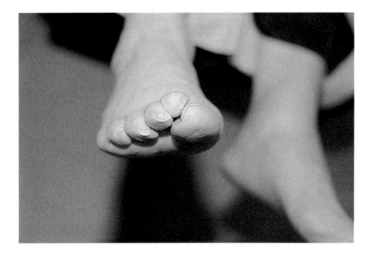

Figure 9.14
Overriding second toe. Involution can be seen in the hallux nail plate.

shoe can reflect pressure back, causing further nail changes (Figure 9.14).

Hallux rigidus is another common condition in which there is reduction in the range of motion at the first metatarsophalangeal joint. It is characterized by enlargement of the first metatarsal head and a general stiffening of the joint; motion is obtained at the nearest functional joint – the interphalangeal joint of the hallux. Over time the distal phalanx becomes permanently dorsiflexed; the nail often protrudes dorsally and is open to trauma from footwear, leading to possible onychauxis or onychocryptosis (Figure 9.15).

Problems with the lesser digits can also adversely affect the nail apparatus (Figure 9.16); these can be congenital or acquired. Frequently affected are feet with the second toe longer than the first, which can lead to the longer toe suffering increased trauma from the end of a shoe or by stubbing and secondary onychomycosis. Longer toes may suffer trauma in the shoe, leading to subungual haematoma and consequent long-term changes in the nail structure.

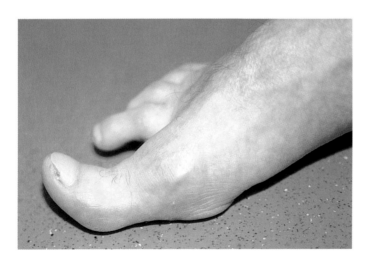

Figure 9.15
Hallux rigidus with compensatory hyperextension of the distal phalanx. Early onychocryptosis is evident.

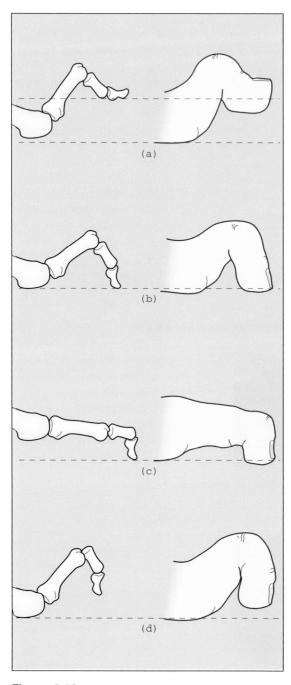

Figure 9.16
Various lesser digit deformities commonly seen in the foot, which may cause nail dystrophy. (a) hammer; (b) claw; (c) mallet; (d) retracted toe.

Other digital deformities of the lesser toes arise as a consequence of footwear, trauma, disease or abnormal foot function. During locomotion, rectus alignment of the toes is required during heel lift to permit the long extensors of the anterior leg group to raise the foot for propulsion. Intrinsic muscles of the foot are vital for normal digital alignment and are easily disturbed by excessive pronation and supination, along with diseases that may affect the nerves innervating them, such as diabetes or poliomyelitis. Consequently during gait the toes become destabilized and adopt various deformities.

Footwear

In older age groups, chronic foot disorders are far more prevalent in women. In part this is attributable to footwear and fashion. A UK study of 9-year-old children's feet found that 25% of girls compared with 1% of boys wear unsuitable shoes, notably with a too narrow toe box. Improper fitting often continues into adult life, with women consistently wearing shoes that are 'smaller than their feet'. Assessment of the footwear should help to establish causes of traumatic nail dystrophies. In order to do this, it is important to assess the shoes that the patient wears most often and not those just worn to the consultation! The main causes of nail problems include:

• poor fitting of footwear
• inadequate footwear design or construction
• excessive wear to shoes.

When looking at shoe fit, areas of prime importance are:

1 Heel height – generally if heels are too high, the foot is forced forward into the toe box with every step, traumatizing the anterior part of the foot, especially around the nail apparatus and apices. The higher

the heel, the more damage is likely to occur. It has been the experience of the authors that heel heights greater than 30–35 mm can yield unwanted effects.

2   Lack of a suitable fastening – a foot in a shoe without adequate fastening suffers in that the foot is free to move unrestrained in the shoe and inevitably (as with high heels) it tends to slip forward into the toe box region of the shoe, traumatizing the distal aspect. Laces are by far the best method of fastening a shoe. The higher the laces come up from the front of the shoe, the more restraint and support is given to the foot. With patients who, because of arthritis, cannot reach or tie laces, Velcro straps make a reasonable substitute.

3   Poor toe box design – in order to restrict rubbing and other trauma to the forefoot and nails, a good toe box is a vital feature. Adequate depth and width ensure no undue pressure is placed on the digital areas (Figure 9.17); allied with a suitable fastening this ensures that the foot stays well back from the tip of the shoe and into the heel. Modern shoes are still produced with inadequate width or depth in the toe box area. One can often see the effects of this when toe outlines are visible from the outside of the shoe. It is wise to feel inside the upper of the shoe; one can often feel a dent or a tear in the lining corresponding to the affected digit. The nail itself can give other clues. A nail with unusual pigmentation may

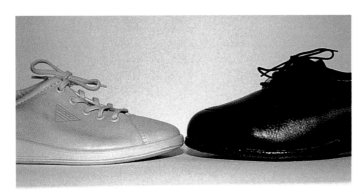

(a)

Figure 9.17
(a) Shoes positioned tip to tip, to demonstrate difference in toe box depths. (b) Shallow toe box design contributes to nail problems: a subungual haematoma due to pressure and rubbing from the shoe toe box.

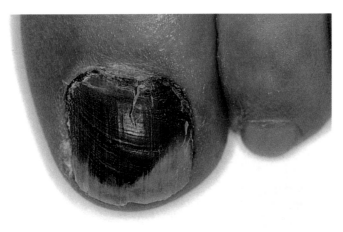

(b)

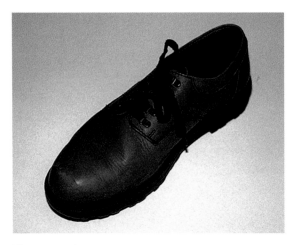

Figure 9.18
A seamless fronted shoe.

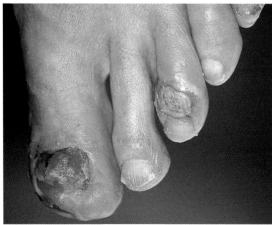

Figure 9.19
Nail unit injury in a diabetic patient with severe vascular disease; this injury was caused by the swift removal of a sticking plaster.

have acquired this from rubbing on the leather of new shoes. More commonly, though, a single toe nail with a highly polished sheen is the result of continuous rubbing on the soft upper of a shoe.

4 Seams that run over the toe box region of the shoe to give an aesthetic touch can be the cause of problems. Inside the shoe, the stitching producing the seam may be readily felt in the shoe upper, impinging on the toe area; such stitching is best avoided (Figure 9.18).

5 Shoes that are too long or without a suitable fastening (slip-on) can often lead to increased nail trauma as, to compensate for the excessive movement, toes become clawed to maintain ground contact and increase stability.

Other factors

When looking at causative factors of nail problems one must always consider the patients' circumstances. Toe nail problems in the aged can be particularly distressing. Not only are they complicated by reduced circulation and sensation, with all the dangers to the foot that this can entail (Figure 9.19), but poor eyesight and decreased manual dexterity in the elderly patient contribute to nail management difficulties. In addition, reduced mobility in the joints of the lower extremity makes it difficult to reach the foot for nail care.

The amount of time a person spends on their feet may affect the severity of the nail problem. Moreover, the footwear worn during these periods will be crucial. Occupational footwear is notorious for precipitating such problems. Occlusive footwear worn for long periods can lead to the retention of excessive perspiration (Figure 9.20). This may predispose to skin infection, which in time, may go on to affect the nail and surrounding tissues. This is often seen in manual workers whose job entails wearing rubber or plastic boots. The transportation and construction industries provide the highest incidence of foot injuries. Since the introduction of steel toe-cap shoes

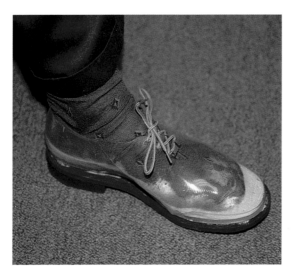

Figure 9.20
A clear shoe showing the extent of perspiration.

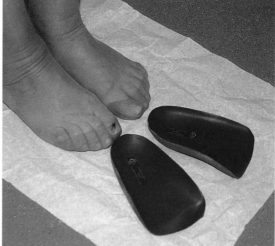

Figure 9.21
Various orthoses which may correct abnormal foot function and digital alignment.

the incidence has been reduced, but even these are not without their problems. The rigidity of the toe box has meant that incorrectly fitting boots have led to toe and nail injuries as a result of their design.

Reducing microtrauma to the nail unit

In order to reduce pressures across the digital areas various orthopaedic devices may be used. Where foot mechanics are considered to be the cause, functional orthoses may be prescribed to control excessive pronatory forces and prevent deterioration (Figures 9.21–9.23). Changes in footwear style are also often advisable. In addition local digital pressures may be reduced by the use of cushioning insoles to reduce repeated microtrauma. Silicone digital appliances may be used to correct or realign digits and so relieve abnormal forces around the nail unit.

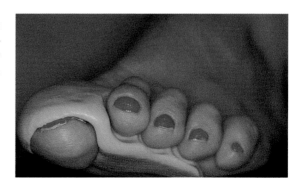

Figure 9.22

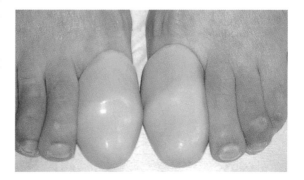

Figure 9.23

Alteration to surrounding tissue

Subungual haemorrhage

Tennis (or sportman's) toe is a brown–black discoloration due to subungual haemorrhage caused by special stresses on the longest toe (great toe and/or the second toe). Pain is associated with the appearance of the damage. In tennis, this occurs because the player frequently stops abruptly; the forward motion of the body propels the toes into the toe box and tip of the footwear. Hard playing surfaces contribute to the injury.

In distinction to tennis toe, jogger's toe tends to involve the third, fourth and fifth toes, apparently due to the constant pounding of the foot on the running surface. The process begins with erythema, oedema and onycholysis or subungual haemorrhage. Throbbing pain often accompanies this condition. Secondary infection resulting in cellulitis and abscess formation may be a rare complication.

Hyperkeratotic changes

Any abnormal intermittent pressure is likely to lead to the development of hyperkeratosis. Typical predisposing factors include:

- abnormal gait or foot mechanics
- poor fitting footwear
- bony deformity.

Corns and callosity

Callosity (callus) develops as a result of intermittent shear and pressure leading to a characteristic yellow thickening of the stratum corneum. Callus on the digits develops most commonly on the lateral side of the fifth toe in women as a result of tight footwear. Where toes are hammer or clawed in shape, apical callus may also develop, and may extend proximally under the nail plate (Figure 9.24).

Corns (heloma, clavus) are the next stage of callus development. Continued pressure results in a sharply demarcated area of hyperkeratosis with a central core or nucleus which protrudes deep into the dermis, causing pain and local inflammation (Figure 9.25). Subungual corns are most commonly observed in the hallux as a result of pressure from footwear, or from a nail or toe deformity such as involution. Typically, lesions develop in the lateral nail sulci or along the distal nail edge (Figure 9.26). As the lesion develops subungually local onycholysis is seen with a subtle yellow discoloration of the detaching nail plate. At this stage differentiation is required from a subungual exostosis or other

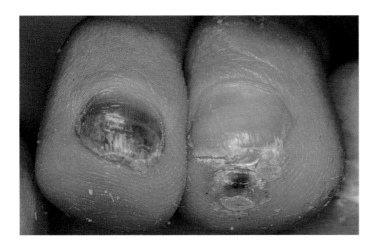

Figure 9.24
Apical corn (heloma). These lesions often extend proximally under the nail plate.

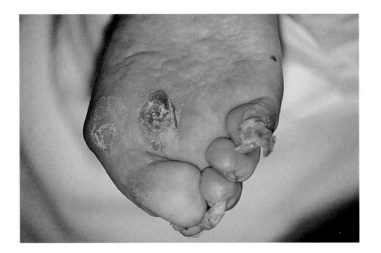

Figure 9.25
Hyperkeratosis due to footwear
and neglect. A large corn can be
seen adjacent to the fifth nail.
(Courtesy of B. Wing.)

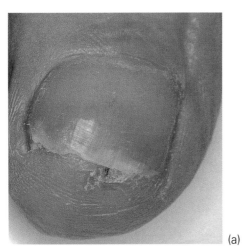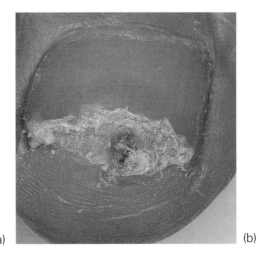

(a)   (b)

Figure 9.26
Subungual
corn: (a) nail
intact; (b)
nail plate
clipped away
to show the
heloma.

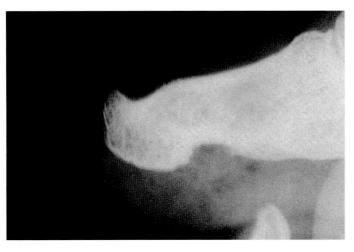

Figure 9.27
Toe X-ray showing a dorsal
hyperostosis.

phalanx abnormality such as tufting (Figure 9.27). Pressure on a subungual corn will lead to blanching, whereas an exostosis offers solid resistance and does not blanch. Radiological imaging is required to establish the diagnosis.

Onychophosis
Corns and callus that develop in the lateral nail folds are termed 'onychophosis'. The condition typically arises as a result of pressure from adjacent or overriding toes, tight footwear, or underlying an involuted nail (Figure 9.28). The condition for many is asymptomatic but frequently it may cause considerable pain when any direct pressure is applied to the distal aspect of the nail plate.

Complications of hyperkeratosis
When the forces of pressure become overwhelming, local haemorrhage or extravasation may appear in the hyperkeratotic tissue

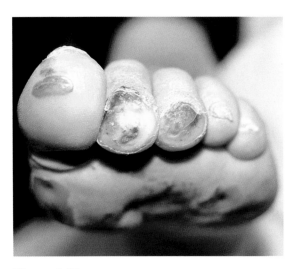

Figure 9.29
Extravasated apical callus, following debridement, in a person with diabetes.

giving a red-brown spotted appearance. This is a sign that ulceration is likely to ensue and therefore requires preventive measures (Figure 9.29).

Treatment of hyperkeratotic changes
When hyperkeratotic changes around the nail give rise to symptoms, immediate treatment involves conservative resection of the nail plate to expose the lesion. Hyperkeratosis can then be debrided by a scalpel. Stubborn sulcal callus may benefit from hydrogen peroxide solution applied to it prior to treatment. Where the overlying nail is thickened or deformed, reduction of the nail by drilling may be required and nail edges should be filed well back (Figure 9.30). Following resection, packing the nail sulci lightly with cotton wool may reduce discomfort.

Preventive measures include the regular application of urea-based emollients to the nail sulci to soften the surrounding skin. Footwear should also be assessed and appropriate advice should be given. Where possible overlapping toes or other causative digital

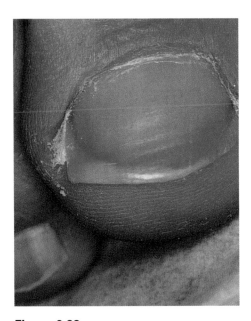

Figure 9.28
Painful lateral hyperkeratosis (from repeated microtrauma) – onychophosis.

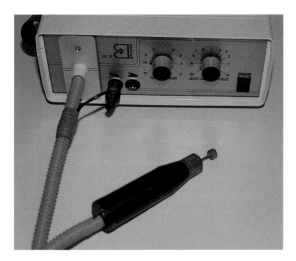

Figure 9.30
An electric nail drill with diamond burr.

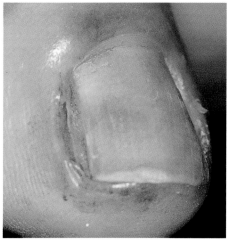

Figure 9.31
Traumatic onycholysis following bulla
formation.

deformities may be accommodated and
protected by the use of silicone appliances.

Onycholysis and onychomadesis

Excess friction between the nail and the shoe
may result in onycholysis and even in fluid-
filled blisters. These subungual bullae can
sometimes be haemorrhagic (Figure 9.31).
Similar friction at the base of the nail may
produce onychomadesis. Separation of the nail
from the subungual tissue is often seen in
ballet dancers who dance on 'points' and in
footballers. Subungual hyperkeratosis is
usually associated with excessive pressure
and related onycholysis, and occasionally
onychomycosis, especially in the elderly.
Overlapping of the second toe on the lateral
aspect of the hallux may also produce onycholysis in this area with or without haemorrhage
(Figure 9.32). Careful examination of the toe
box of the regular footwear may reveal bulging
or tearing of the leather internally when
footwear is at fault.

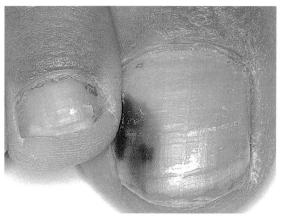

Figure 9.32
'Primary' onycholysis due to pressure from the
second toe.

Onychocryptosis

Onychocryptosis is the term applied when the
nail plate embeds, to varying degrees, into the
periungual tissues. Four types can be
described in adults:

- juvenile ingrowing toe nail
- hypertrophy of the lateral lip
- pincer or involuted nail
- distal nail embedding.

Juvenile ingrowing toe nail (subcutaneous ingrowing nail)

Ingrowing toe nail is created by impingement of the nail plate onto the dermal tissue of the lateral nail fold. This often results from improper trimming of the nail. Consequently, a lacerating spicule of the nail pierces the soft tissue surrounding the side of the nail, acting as a foreign body and producing inflammation with pain from perforation of the nail groove epithelium.

Juvenile ingrowing toe nail (Figure 9.33) is most frequently observed in the hallux of

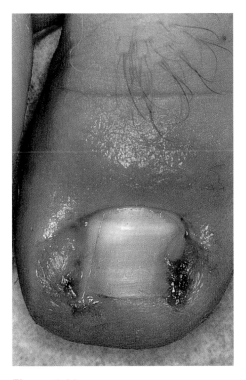

Figure 9.33
Ingrowing toe nail with chronic granulation tissue formation.

adolescents, rarely seen in the lesser digits. The relatively thin nail plate, in combination with hyperhidrosis softening the surrounding skin, promotes the development of the condition. Bilateral cases are common, particularly where there is a family history of ingrowing nails.

Conservative treatment, with or without local anaesthesia, in mild cases consists of resection of the offending nail spike using nail clippers or a scalpel blade. Once the nail fragment has been retrieved, the nail edge should be filed smooth. In some cases cotton wool packing may prevent further trauma from the nail plate on the affected sulci. Any local infection should be treated with the appropriate systemic antibiotics. Subsequently the patient should be advised with regard to proper nail care to prevent recurrence. Unfortunately, as conservative management requires a high degree of compliance, recurrences are frequent. Sometimes, the nail groove becomes involved along its entire length by excess granulation tissue which may extend beneath the nail and overlap its dorsal aspect.

The definitive treatment procedure calls for selective matrix horn removal, under local anaesthesia, which permanently narrows the nail (Figure 9.34). A nail elevator is used to free a lateral nail strip down to the proximal nail fold, nail bed and matrix. Nail nippers are then used to cut the nail vertically along its length to the matrix, under the eponychium. Locking forceps are applied to the separated nail section and medially rotated until the section is freed. The area is then washed with saline and cleared of any debris prior to a 3-minute application of liquefied phenol. This is applied and worked into the exposed nail matrix and nail bed using a Black's file or similar instrument. The area is then carefully dried and dressed. Postoperative pain is minimal since phenol has local anaesthetic action and is also antiseptic. The matrix epithelium is sloughed off and there is usually slight oozing for 2–4

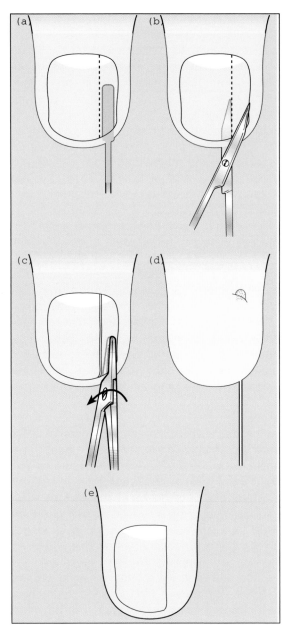

Figure 9.34
Nail wedge resection procedure. (a) nail edge is elevated; (b) nail is cut using Thwaite nipper; (c) forceps are attached and the section of nail is medial rotated; (d) Liquid phenol solution is applied for 3 minutes; (e) end result following resolution.

weeks. Daily footbaths with hypertonic saline minimize the risk of infection and assist healing.

Hypertrophy of the lateral lip
Hypertrophic lateral nail fold usually accompanies long-standing ingrowing toe nail deformities. The nail looks normal or slightly involuted, but a soft tissue lip overgrows around the edge of a nail plate and onychophosis may develop in the affected sulcus (Figure 9.35). The hypertrophic lip usually forms along the fibular sulcus of the hallux as a result of the adjacent second toe impinging upon it, rolling the flesh around the nail plate. Hypertrophic lips on the tibial sulcus of the hallux occur often as a result of abnormal locomotor forces secondary to toe deformities such as hallux valgus and hallux rigidus.

Where toe impingement is a problem, silicone interdigital wedges may reduce symptoms (Figure 9.36). Surgical treatment consists of narrowing the nail by cauterization of the lateral horn of the nail matrix, as for juvenile ingrowing toe nail. Complete removal of the affected part of the nail and the hypertrophic lateral nail fold may be achieved by the Winograd procedure (Figure 9.37). Using a double incisional technique an entire wedge of nail plate, matrix and nail fold is removed down to bone and the remaining edges are brought together with sutures. This procedure is also occasionally used to treat juvenile ingrowing toe nails, when faster healing times are required.

Pincer nail (trumpet nail, omega nail, involuted nail)
Pincer nail is a dystrophy characterized by transverse overcurvature increasing along the longitudinal axis of the nail and reaching its greatest extent at the distal part. The edges constrict the nail bed tissue and dig into the lateral nail grooves. Pain is usually not too severe but may sometimes be excruciating, and onychophosis may be present. On

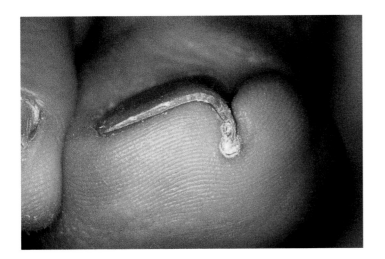

Figure 9.35
Hypertrophy of the lateral lip (nail fold).

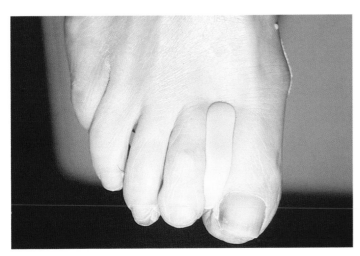

Figure 9.36
Silicone interdigital wedge, preventing pressure of the fibular sulcus of the hallux.

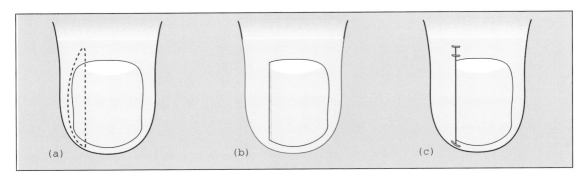

Figure 9.37
The Winograd procedure. (a) tissue for excision (b) a 'D' shaped incision is made including the nail matrix and overlying soft tissues (c) post-operative appearance .

occasion, pain may develop specifically under the midpoint of the distal nail edge, dorsal to the distal phalangeal tuft. Two varieties of overcurvature can be described:

1 Symmetrical involvement of several toes, usually with lateral deviation of the long axis of the hallux nail and medial deviation of the lesser toe nails (Figure 9.38). This variety is probably genetically determined. The pincer nail syndrome includes gryphosis of finger and toe nails in combination with acro-osteolytic shortening of the terminal phalanx and destructive arthrosis

of the distal joints of the digits. An X-ray examination reveals a wider base of the terminal phalanx, often with lateral osteophytes. Hyperostosis is frequently observed on the dorsal tuft of the distal phalanx, due to traction of the heaped-up nail bed which is firmly attached to the bone by collagen fibres.

2 Asymmetrical involvement of the halluces, the major cause being foot deformities and osteoarthritis (Figure 9.39).

Conservative management is suitable for mild to moderate deformity, which may be

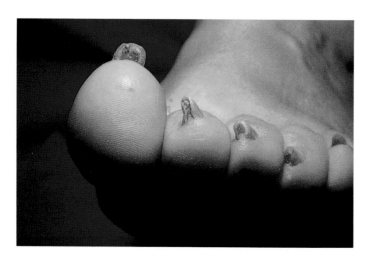

Figure 9.38
Pincer nail deformity with symmetrical involvement of several toes.

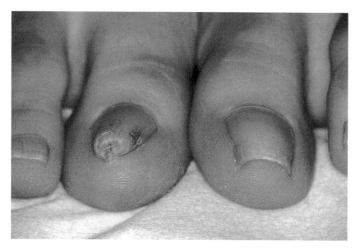

Figure 9.39
Involuted or trumpet nail – often painful.

improved by simple resection of the involuted shoulders of nail with clearance of any underlying onychophosis – relief is usually instant. Any thickening of the nail plate itself can be reduced using a nail drill. Advice should also be given regarding footwear with a deep toe box to eliminate dorsal pressure on the nail.

More severe deformity may benefit from a nail brace technique which is based on maintaining tension on the nail plate with the wire. Fraser's method consists of a brace constructed to fit the curved plate exactly; at one selected point a minute adjustment (a slight bend) is then made to the brace and it is fitted to the plate. As the nail plate is weaker than the stainless wire, the nail plate conforms to the brace. In the months that follow, a series of adjustments are made and almost imperceptibly the curvature decreases. Some improvements to this technique have been suggested, such as the use of brackets adapted on the dorsum of the nail and linked by a rubber band or attachment of a plastic brace on the surface of the nail. In these cases the nail plate is first flattened with an electric nail drill, and pliant braces are stuck transversely on the nail to counteract the overcurvature (Figure 9.40). However, the

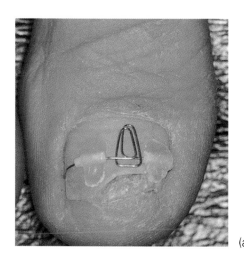

(a)

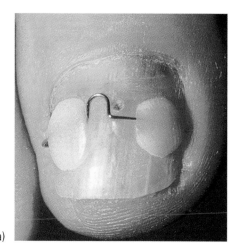

(b)

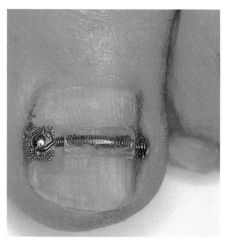

(c)

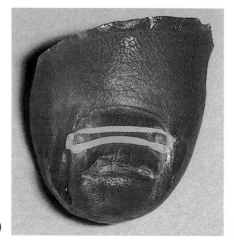

(d)

Figure 9.40
(a–d) Nail brace technique for pincer nail deformity.

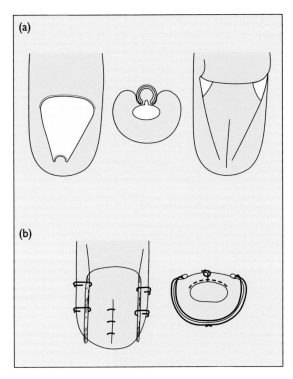

Figure 9.41
(a, b) Haneke's technique for correcton of
pincer nail deformity.

pathogenesis of pincer nail is such that none
of these methods gives a high cure rate.

The definitive procedure is said to be
Haneke's surgical treatment (Figure 9.41): using
a bloodless field, a lateral nail strip involving one
or both sides is freed from the proximal nail fold,
nail bed and matrix with a Freer septum elevator, then cut longitudinally and extracted. This
permits the destruction of the lateral matrix
horns by phenol. The distal two-thirds of the nail
is removed, then a longitudinal median incision
of the nail bed is carried down to the bone. The
entire nail bed is dissected from the phalanx and
the dorsal tuft removed with a bone rongeur. The
nail bed is spread and sutured with 6-0
polydioxanone atraumatic sutures and kept in
this position by reversed tie-over sutures that
pull the lateral nail folds apart; these are left in

for 18–21 days. Daily povidone–iodine antisepsis
prevents infection.

Distal nail embedding

In the great toe, a distal wall may develop after
nail shedding following subungual haemorrhage, for example in tennis toe or after nail
avulsion (Figure 9.42). Normally, the nail plate
position counteracts the forces that are
exerted during walking. Owing to lack of
counterpressure, the plantar portion of the
hallux pulp becomes distorted dorsally when
the foot rolls up and the body weight presses
on the tip of the great toe during walking. The
distal wall interferes with the growth of the
newly formed nail. The anchoring of an acrylic
sculptured nail on the stump nail may enable
it to overgrow the heaped-up distal tissue
(Figure 9.43). Should this procedure not be
effective a crescent-shaped wedge excision
becomes necessary (Figure 9.44). A 'fish

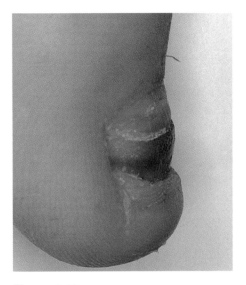

Figure 9.42
Distal nail embedding – overgrowth of distal
soft tissue after nail loss. New nail may
penetrate into this.

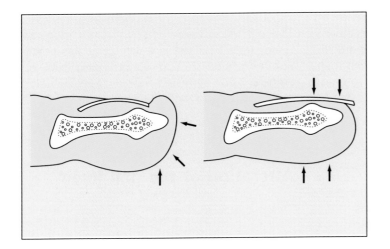

Figure 9.43
Anchoring of acrylic sculptured
nail to inhibit embedding.

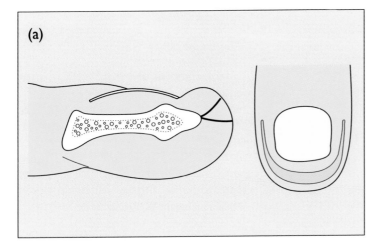

Figure 9.44
(a, b) Removal of overgrown
distal soft tissue.

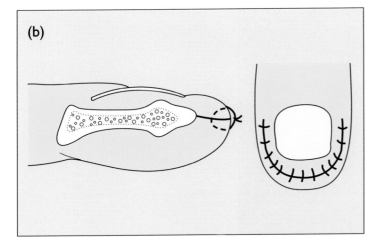

mouth' incision is carried out parallel to the distal groove around the tip of the toe, starting and ending 3–5 mm proximal to the end of the lateral nail fold. A second incision is then made to yield a wedge of 4–8 mm at its greatest width; it has to be dissected from the bone.

Hangnails

Hangnails often result from self-inflicted trauma. Usually limited to the hands, these consist of a small portion of horny epidermis that has split away from the lateral nail fold. They can be painful and lead to secondary bacterial infection. Although frequently found in nail biters, they can also arise from other forms of injury. Cuticle biting and picking may result in recurrent attacks of paronychia.

Paronychia of the toes

Inflammation of the nail folds is common in athletes and is characterized by swelling, erythema, pain and purulent discharge. It is often caused by pressure from the shoe or by secondary infection from ingrowing toe nail. The big toe is more often affected than the lesser toes. Turf toe is a variant of this condition described in competitors who play on artificial turf surfaces; rarely, they develop painful erythema and swelling, mainly of the great toe.

Alteration of the nail itself

This category includes:

1 Self-inflicted injury (Figures 9.45–9.47):
   • the habit of pushing back the cuticle (see Chapter 2)
   • Heller's median nail dystrophy (see Chapter 2)
   • nail biting and picking
   • self-inflicted nail damage – may cause longitudinal melanonychia (LM)
   • nail artefacts, caused by deliberate acts of injury to the nail apparatus with the intention of creating a 'diversion for personal gain'; they may also be caused 'subconsciously'. Nail artefacts take various forms. Such patients usually have psychological problems.

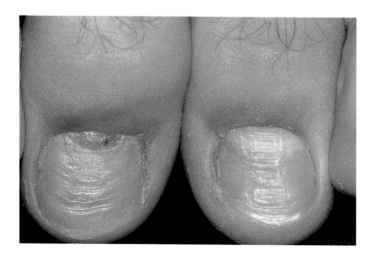

Figure 9.45
Self-induced transverse ridges/furrows.

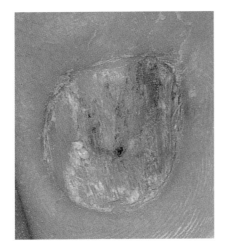

Figure 9.46
Onychotillomania of the great toe.

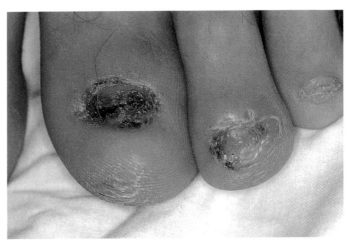

Figure 9.47
Nail dystrophy – self-damage.

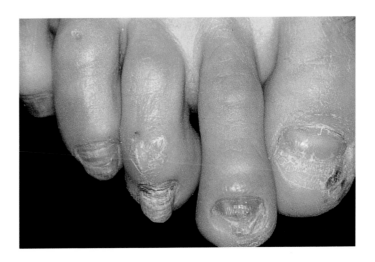

Figure 9.48
Nail shedding in a long-distance runner.

2 Nail shedding (Figure 9.48):
- self-inflicted anonychia of the toe nails is associated with small or absent nails and crushing due to traumatic bleeding
- periodic shedding of the nails can result from biomechanical causes and is frequently seen in runners.

3 Worn-down nail (Figures 9.49, 9.50) (see Chapter 2):
- koilonychia (toes of rickshaw pullers)

4 Brittle nails (see Chapter 6).

5 Onychogryphosis and hypertrophic nail (see Chapter 4).

6 Frictional melanonychia (Figure 9.51):
- frictional melanonychia of the toes can be initiated by repeated trauma from footwear
- friction and pressure are responsible for LM with pseudo-Hutchinson's sign in boxers.

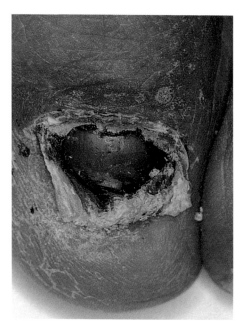

Figure 9.49
Dystrophy due to chronic shoe rubbing.

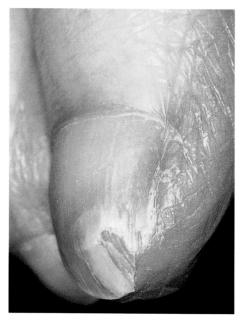

Figure 9.50
Dystrophy from shoe pressure.

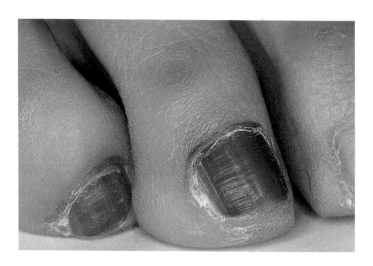

Figure 9.51
Frictional melanonychia.

7 Multiple transverse leukonychia (Figure 9.52). Multiple transverse white bands separated by normal pink nail and paralleling the distal shape of the lunula result from repeated microtrauma. These appear in patients with marked visible free margins of the involved toe nails (usually the great toe or the second toe when longer), indicating a lack of trimming and impinging on the distal part of the shoe.

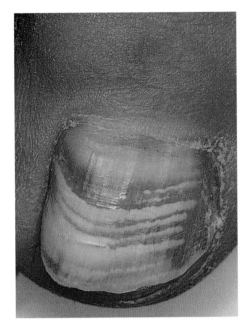

Figure 9.52
Transverse leukonychia from distal pressure on untrimmed nail.

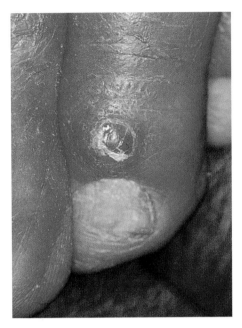

Figure 9.53
Myxoid cyst associated with distal interphalangeal joint osteoarthritis.

Alteration of the bony phalanx

Exostosis can be observed in ballet dancers and football players (see p. 174).

Alteration of the distal joint and tendon sheath

Mucous pseudocyst (Figure 9.53) can be caused by systemic conditions that affect joints and in particular the distal joint (see p. 178). This tumour can produce pressure on the nail matrix resulting in a longitudinal nail groove. When the second toe is longer than the other toes, it may cause increased pressure on the toe from the shoes, especially in tennis players. Treatment usually consists of removal of the cyst and overlying skin and debridement of the arthritic distal interphalangeal joint. Magnetic resonance imaging (MRI) demonstrates the relationship of the cyst to the other soft tissue structures of the toe (Figure 9.54).

THE PAINFUL NAIL

Pain is a non-specific and common symptom of many conditions of the nail apparatus (Table 9.1; Figures 9.55–9.61). Apart from various forms of trauma, many inflammatory and vascular diseases may cause pain; however, pain is so subjective and inconstant a symptom that even diseases commonly known as being particularly painful may follow a rather asymptomatic course and vice versa. The entire distal phalanx, especially the finger

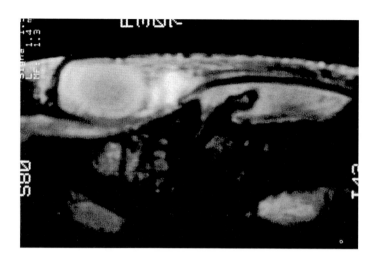

Figure 9.54
Magnetic resonance image
showing myxoid pseudocyst in a
second toe nail in relation to
other soft tissue structures.
(Courtesy of A. Salon, Paris.)

Table 9.1 Causes of painful nail

Trauma
  Childhood malalignment
  Cold injury
  Common type
  Crush and squeeze injuries
  Ingrowing toe nail
  Splinters, foreign bodies
  Sports and sport shoe injuries

Inflammation
  Acro-osteolysis
  Acute (and chronic) paronychia
  Dorsolateral fissures
  Gout
  Herpes simplex
  Implantation epidermoid cyst
  Osteomyelitis
  Pincer nail (severe form enclosing bone)
  Post-cryosurgery (may be prolonged
    bone pain)
  Prosector's wart (tuberculosis)
  Sarcoid dactylitis
  Subcutaneous abscess
  Subungual foreign body
  Ventral pterygium

Tumours (soft tissue and bone)
  Aneurysmal bone cyst
  Bowen's disease
  Enchondroma
  Fibroma
  Glomus tumour
  Keratoacanthoma
  Leiomyoma
  Metastases
  Myxoid cyst
  Osteoid osteoma
  Osteoma, exostosis
  Secondary infection – slow-growing tumour
  Some neuromas
  Squamous cell carcinoma
  Subungual corn
  Subungual papilloma – incontinentia pigmenti
  Subungual wart

Vascular
  Acute ischaemia
  Chilblains
  Raynaud's phenomenon/disease
  Rheumatoid vasculitic lesions
  Systemic sclerosis

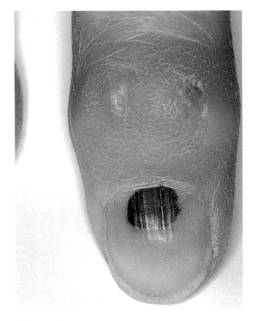

Figure 9.55
Recurrent herpes simplex with
subungual haemorrhage.

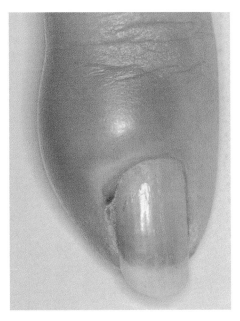

Figure 9.56
Acute paronychia.

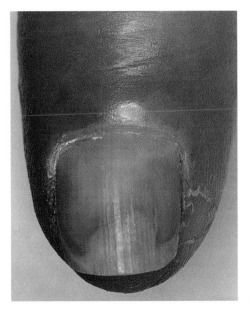

(a)

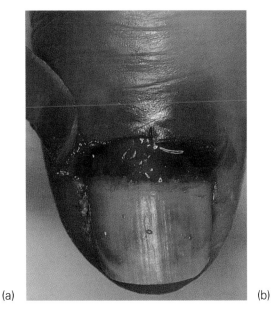

(b)

Figure 9.57
(a) Acute paronychia with pus tracking into the nail bed; (b) treatment by transverse section of the
nail plate.

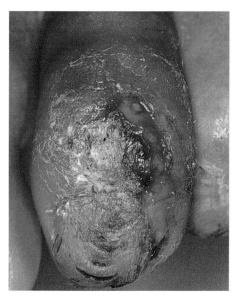

Figure 9.58
Radiodermatitis and radionecrosis of the bony
phalanx following treatment of epidermal
carcinoma.

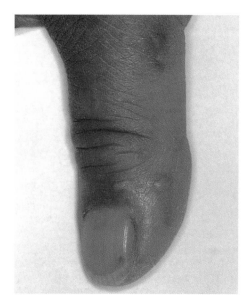

Figure 9.59
Herpes zoster.

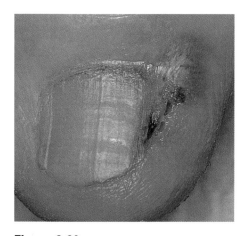

Figure 9.60
Glomus tumour.

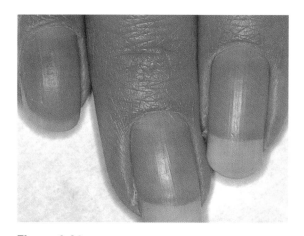

Figure 9.61
Implantation cyst following surgical treatment
for ingrowing toe nail.

pulp, is richly innervated. Each 'space-occupy-
ing' process, whether inflammatory or neoplas-
tic, may produce pain because the subungual
tissue consists of dense fibrous tissue closely
adherent to the bone and without the 'elastic'
pad of subcutaneous fat. Inflammatory conditions and tumours are squeezed in this firm
subungual tissue between the hard nail plate

and hard bone; slowly enlarging processes may lead to clubbing and pressure-induced bone erosion. Pain is therefore to be expected under these conditions. In addition, the tumour itself may be inherently painful, as for example with the glomus tumour. If pain subsequent to simple trauma or acute inflammation does not respond to adequate therapy, either an X-ray or biopsy or both should be performed to rule out a malignant tumour. Radiographs may be difficult to interpret, especially in the elderly with degenerative arthritis, and it may be necessary to repeat the X-rays or other imaging techniques if the disease does not follow the expected course, or fails to respond to treatment. Ultrasound and MRI may be useful tools but the latter is very expensive.

FURTHER READING

Balkin SW (1993) What do women want: comfy shoes – sometimes, *JMA* **269**: 215.

Baran R (1987) Frictional longitudinal melanonychia: a new entity, *Dermatologica* **174**: 280–284.

Baran R (1990) Nail biting and picking as a possible cause of longitudinal melanonychia, *Dermatologica* **181**: 126–128.

Baran R (1995) Transverse leuconychia of toe nails due to repeated microtrauma, *Br J Dermatol* **133**: 267–269.

Baran R, Badillet G (1982) Primary onycholysis of the big toe nail: review of 113 cases, *Br J Dermatol* **106**: 529–534.

Bayerl C, Moll I (1993) Longitudinal melanonychia with Hutchinson's sign in a boxer, *Hautarzt* **44**: 476–479.

Dagnall C (1976) The development of nail treatments, *Br J Chiropody* **41**: 206–207.

Dawber RPR, Bristow I, Turner W (2001) *A Text Atlas of Podiatric Dermatology* (London, Martin Dunitz).

Doller J, Strother S (1978) Turf toe, *J Am Podiatr Assoc* **68**: 512–514.

Effendy I, Ossowski B, Happle R (1993) Zangennagel, *Hautarzt* **44**: 800–802.

Eiscle SA (1994) Conditions of the toe nails, *Orthop Clin North Am* **25**: 183–187.

Fabry H (1983) Haut- und Nagelveränderungen bei Hallux valgus, *Akt Derm* **9**: 77–79.

Gibbs RC (1985) Toenail disease secondary to poorly fitting shoes or abnormal biomechanics, *Cutis* **36**: 399–400.

Gibbs RC, Boxer MC (1989) Abnormal biomechanics of feet and their cause of hyperkeratoses, *J Am Acad Dermatol* **6**: 1061–1069.

Haneke E, Baran R (1994) In: *Nail Surgery and Traumatic Abnormalities*, eds Baran R, Dawber RPR (Oxford, Blackwell Scientific), pp. 344–415.

Helphand AE (1989) Nail and hyperkeratotic problems in the elderly foot, *AFP* **39**: 101–110.

Hurley PT, Balu V (1982) Self inflicted anonychia, *Arch Dermatol* **118**: 956–957.

Jahss MH (1979) Geriatric aspects of the foot and ankle. In: *Clinical Geriatrics*, ed. Rossman I (Philadelphia, JB Lippincott) pp. 638–650.

Johnson EW In Tarara EL (1970) Ingrown toe nail: a problem among the aged, *Post Grad Med* **••**: 199–202.

O'Toole EA, Stephens R, Young MM *et al* (1995) Subungual melanoma: a relation to direct injury? *J Am Acad Dermatol* **33**: 525–528.

Price MA, Bruce S, Waidhofer W *et al* (1994) Beau's lines and pyogenic granulomas following hand trauma, *Cutis* **54**: 246–249.

Rzonca EC, Lupo PJ (1989) Pedal nail pathology: biomechanical implications, *Clin Podiatr Med Surg* **6**: 327–337.

Scher RK (1978) Jogger's toe, *Int J Dermatol* **17**: 719–720.

Singh D, Bentley G, Trevino SG (1996) Callosities, corns and calluses, *Br Med J* **312**: 1403–1406

Stone OJ, Mullins JF (1963) The distal course of nail matrix hemorrhage, *Arch Dermatol* **88**: 186.

Zook EG (1986) Complications of the perionychium, *Hand Clin* **2**: 407–427.

10 Histopathology of common nail conditions

Eckart Haneke

Onychomycosis • Psoriasis • Pityriasis rubra pilaris • Lichen planus • Lupus erythematosus • Alopecia areata • Eczema • Parakeratosis pustulosa • Pemphigus and pemphigoid • Dyskeratosis follicularis and benign pemphigus • Amyloidosis • Digital herpes simplex • Hand, foot and mouth disease • Tumours and reactive tumorous lesions • Further reading

Nail disorders are rarely subjected to thorough histopathological investigation. In contrast to skin, the nail is not easy to biopsy and many physicians as well as patients are therefore reluctant to undertake this procedure. To obtain relevant results it is necessary to consider the following:

1 Nail changes usually reflect a pathological process of the matrix or (much less frequently) of the nail bed. The biopsy must contain a relevant piece of matrix.
2 Some changes that are obvious to the naked eye may almost be invisible in a microscopic section. This is not infrequently the case in nail pigmentations (see Chapter 7).
3 Nail clippings are useful for the diagnosis of onychomycosis and a few other conditions. However, as in routine mycology, subungual keratotic material usually harbours the greatest amount of fungal elements.
4 The nail organ often reacts differently from normal epidermis.
5 Nail specimens are difficult to handle and process in the histopathological laboratory.

Tears and folds are the rule rather than the exception.

There are particular reaction patterns that differ in the nail from those of common epidermis:

- A granular layer is always pathological in the matrix and nail bed and leads to onycholysis.
- Irritation that would cause parakeratosis in the epidermis often induces pathological orthokeratinization.
- Spongiosis is often seen in disorders that would not cause spongiosis in skin, e.g. in psoriasis or lichen planus.
- Changes in the nail plate are most often non-specific; they may suggest a diagnosis but do not provide proof.

ONYCHOMYCOSIS

Fungal infections of the nail organ are the most common nail disorders. Even though they are usually easily diagnosable they may be indistinguishable from nail psoriasis and the conditions may in fact occur together.

Superficial white onychomycosis is easy to diagnose: a tangential biopsy of the nail plate is taken with a no. 15 scalpel and sent to the laboratory. Formalin fixation is not necessary. The thin nail slice is processed and cut as usual and stained with periodic acid–Schiff reagent (PAS) or another stain for fungi. Under the microscope, chains of small, regularly sized fungal spores are seen on the nail plate surface and in its splits, giving evidence of a *Trichophyton mentagrophytes* infection. Larger spores and short, thick-walled hyphae of irregular calibre are characteristic of a mould infection. The nail plate does not exhibit any further pathological alterations and the subungual structures remain normal.

Endonyx onychomycosis can be diagnosed by examining nail clippings. Usually due to *T. soudanense*, it shows a dense infiltration of the nail substance with relatively thin hyphae.

To diagnose distal and distal lateral subungual onychomycosis, either nail clippings with adherent subungual hyperkeratosis or a nail biopsy are necessary. Clipped material shows variable amounts of irregular masses of hyphae and often also thick-walled arthrospores. In addition, the subungual keratotic material may contain small, dried neutrophilic abscesses and serum globules that are also PAS positive and may be mistaken for fungal elements if very small. Nail biopsies reveal important pathological alterations of the nail bed and matrix with subepithelial lymphocytic infiltrates, spongiosis, lymphocytic exocytosis and intraepithelial neutrophils, which often form Munro's microabscesses in the keratin just beneath the nail plate. If there are only few fungi the wrong diagnosis of psoriasis unguium may then be made. The nail plate's undersurface may be invaded by hyphae, which usually are seen in a longitudinal and parallel arrangement. This is proof that the affected nail is still growing normally.

For the diagnosis of proximal subungual onychomycosis, a disc of nail plate may be punched out of the nail plate; this is best done after soaking the digit in water for 10 minutes, to soften the nail plate. The punch is carefully advanced through the entire thickness of the nail plate until the reactive subungual keratosis is reached. The tissue sample is embedded, cut, and stained for fungi. In onychomycoses hyphae are seen to penetrate the entire thickness of the nail plate. Nail biopsies that include the proximal nail fold, nail plate, matrix and nail bed show hyphae in the stratum corneum of the underside of the proximal nail fold as well as fungi in different levels of the nail plate. Inflammatory changes are not pronounced as long as the fungi have not reached the nail bed epithelium.

Total dystrophic onychomycosis shows variably severe changes. An intact nail plate is no longer seen, being replaced by irregular keratotic debris containing large amounts of fungal elements, both spores and hyphae. The latter are arranged in a haphazard fashion. The keratin contains also neutrophils and neutrophilic abscesses. The matrix and nail bed often exhibit papillomatosis and pronounced spongiosis. There is a considerable oedema in the papillary dermis and a variably dense lymphocytic infiltrate.

PSORIASIS

Nail psoriasis is most commonly characterized by pits, 'salmon' or oil patches, onycholysis and nail dystrophy. Pits develop from tiny psoriatic lesions located in the most proximal matrix region. These produce parakeratotic mounds which remain on the nail plate surface as long as the growing nail is covered by the proximal nail fold; they then break off and leave a small depression in the nail surface. The depth of the pits reflects the severity of the lesion, their longitudinal diameter their duration. Salmon spots are psoriatic lesions in the distal matrix or nail bed. There is an inflammatory, mainly lymphocytic infiltrate in the upper dermis with wide capillaries, mild to moderate spongiosis with lymphocytic exocytosis and parakeratosis that may contain single neutrophils or small neutrophilic abscesses. Serum imbibition of the parakeratosis is probably the cause of their yellowish colour. When such a lesion reaches the hyponychium air penetrates under the nail plate and onycholysis develops. Psoriatic leukonychia is characterised by a more or less circumscribed area of parakeratosis in the nail plate. Splinter haemorrhages represent thrombosed, ectatic psoriatic capillaries.

Acrodermatitis continua suppurative of Hallopeau may show different lesions: alterations known from pustular psoriasis, a spongiotic variant, or both spongiform pustules and spongiotic vesicles.

Reiter's disease essentially exhibits psoriasiform changes, but the pustular component may be more pronounced and there is usually more erythrocyte extravasation.

PITYRIASIS RUBRA PILARIS

Pityriasis rubra pilaris may rarely involve the nail. It is characterized by subungual hyperkeratosis with alternating ortho- and parakeratosis. An inflammatory infiltrate may be seen in the periungual skin.

LICHEN PLANUS

Lichen planus of the nails usually affects the proximal matrix and undersurface of the proximal nail fold. A dense, band-like lymphocytic infiltrate is seen directly beneath the epidermis or matrix epithelium, respectively. Liquefaction degeneration of basal cells may

be pronounced, causing extensive split formation between the dermis and epithelium. The latter tends to thin out and usually develops hypergranulosis. This in turn does not transform into normal nail substance. Involvement of the most proximal matrix is responsible for the frequent loss of nail sheen. With time, the cul-de-sac where the proximal nail plate is located flattens until it completely disappears and overgrows the matrix with loss of nail formation, which is clinically seen as a pterygium dorsale. Particularly in the matrix and proximal nail bed, spongiosis may be seen and even cause tiny spongiotic vesicles. Bullous nail lichen planus has also been observed.

Lichen striatus shows a band-like dense lymphocytic infiltrate of the affected nail portions with hydropic degeneration of basal cells, exocytosis, mild spongiosis, occasional dyskeratoses and granulosis.

LUPUS ERYTHEMATOSUS

Lupus erythematosus, especially chilblain lupus, may involve finger and toe tips, which become bluish-red to violaceous with considerable nail dystrophy. Histopathological examination shows irregular involvement of the matrix and nail bed. There is a patchy, but usually band-like, dense epidermotropic infiltrate and a thickening of the PAS positive basal membrane zone. Orthokeratotic and parakeratotic keratinization are seen, as well as onycholysis and epithelial atrophy.

ALOPECIA AREATA

Alopecia areata of the nail is essentially a spongiotic dermatitis. The matrix and nail bed show a perivascular, band-like lymphocytic infiltrate that migrates into the spongiotic epithelium. Small spongiotic vesicles containing plasma are transported upwards and included in the nail plate, giving it its characteristic rough, opaque and thickened structure.

ECZEMA

Allergic contact dermatitis (eczema) is microscopically similar to alopecia areata; however, the spongiosis may be more pronounced, leading to gross nail plate irregularities. Particularly in protein contact dermatitis due to food, there may also be a spongiotic dermatitis of the proximal nail fold.

PARAKERATOSIS PUSTULOSA

Parakeratosis pustulosa (Hjorth–Sabouraud syndrome) shows both eczematoid and psoriasiform alterations: mild to dense lymphocytic infiltrates around dilated capillaries of the upper dermis, occasional papillomatosis, spongiosis and exocytosis, spongiotic vesicles and pustulation as well as crust formation.

PEMPHIGUS AND PEMPHIGOID

The autoimmune bullous disorders do not exhibit specific features differentiating them from skin lesions. Pemphigus vulgaris may involve the matrix and nail bed with suprabasal acantholytic cleft formation and subsequent nail thinning. Bullous pemphigoid is characterized by a subepithelial cleft formation and an eosinophil-rich infiltrate. Cicatricial pemphigoid rarely involves the nail and may cause considerable nail dystrophy. Immunofluorescence examinations, sometimes enzyme-linked immunosorbent assay (ELISA), immunoblotting and immunoprecipitation, are necessary to distinguish these dermatoses.

DYSKERATOSIS FOLLICULARIS AND BENIGN PEMPHIGUS

Dyskeratosis follicularis (Darier's disease) often involves the nail with whitish and reddish longitudinal streaks. Histologically, a pronounced subungual hyperkeratosis may be seen with dyskeratoses remaining identifiable. Furthermore, multinucleate epithelial cells, clumping cells and corps ronds are seen. Suprabasal cleft formation may be absent in the nail bed. Benign familiar pemphigus (Hailey–Hailey disease) is very similar, but multinucleate cells are usually not observed.

AMYLOIDOSIS

Dystrophic nails, clinically very similar to nail lichen planus, are characteristic of nail involvement in amyloidosis. Histological investigation reveals amyloid depositions around blood vessels and in the superficial dermis which interfere with nail substance formation. The amyloid exhibits positive Congo red staining and a bright light-green colour under polarization microscopy.

DIGITAL HERPES SIMPLEX

Recurrent herpes simplex – despite being rarely diagnosed – is not infrequent. Any recurrent blistering process around a finger nail, particularly when accompanied by early lymphangitis and radiating pain, should prompt a cytological examination. The blister roof is opened and a Tzanck smear taken for microscopic investigation as well as for virus culture or molecular biological tests. Early blisters with clear watery contents exhibit mainly keratinocytes, some of which are giant and multinucleated. Securing the blister roof for histological sections may be necessary to rule out an early bullous impetigo (run-around).

Herpes zoster infrequently extends to the digits. Tzanck tests demonstrate an essentially similar picture to that of herpes simplex.

HAND, FOOT AND MOUTH DISEASE

Typically, small oval vesicles are seen around the nails with a greyish-white blister roof and a narrow red rim. Histology of early lesions reveals spongiosis, mononuclear exocytosis and an occasional large keratinocyte. Electron microscopy revealed intranuclear Coxsackie viruses.

TUMOURS AND REACTIVE TUMOROUS LESIONS

There is a wide variety of tumours and tumour-like lesions originating from virtually all the different tissue structures found in the tip of a digit: epithelium (epidermal, sweat gland, nail), melanocytes, connective tissue, blood and lymph vessels, nerves, bone, tendon sheath, benign and malignant systemic diseases, and metastases. A few that are rarely seen in other sites are briefly described below.

Keratin cysts

Various types of keratin-filled cysts may occur under or around the nail. Traumatic implantation cysts are lined by epidermis and contain orthokeratin. Intraosseous implantation cysts demonstrate the same histological features.

Nail surgery that displaces matrix and/or nail bed epithelium may give rise to a cyst in which parts of the wall reveal exactly the same structure as a trichilemmal cyst – it might well be called an onycholemmal cyst – and which contains compact eosinophilic keratin distinguishable from epidermal keratin.

Onycholemmal horn

Onycholemmal horn is histologically similar to proliferating trichilemmal tumour. Clinically the lesion has a warty appearance and histologically it consists of an epithelial proliferation with keratinocytes enlarging toward the surface and producing large amounts of keratin containing necrotic keratinocytes. There is no true crater and shoulder formation.

Keratoacanthoma

Keratoacanthoma is a fast-growing, painful lesion usually arising from the hyponychium or the lateral nail groove. In the tip of the digit it exhibits a more vertical growth pattern, rapidly reaching and eroding the bone. A marked lateral lip and keratin-filled crater are characteristic. Suprabasal keratinocytes are large, rich in glycogen, and towards the horn-filled crater often contain keratohyalin granules. Staining for p53, Ki1 and proliferating cell nuclear antigens gives a more regular peripheral staining in keratoacanthoma than in squamous cell carcinoma, but this is not clear-cut enough to make this pattern a differential diagnostic tool.

Distal warty tumours of incontinentia pigmenti

Women with incontinentia pigmenti (Bloch–Sulzberger syndrome) may develop intensely painful subungual keratotic tumours. These tumours represent verrucous hyperplastic papillomatous lesions with granulosis and hyperkeratosis. Dyskeratoses are seen to occur at all levels of the epidermis and in the hyperkeratosis just as in the second stage of incontinentia pigmenti.

Onychomatricoma

Onychomatricoma is a recently described entity, clinically characterized by a thickened, yellow longitudinal nail portion with splinter haemorrhages and a slight overcurvature, consisting of a markedly papillomatous lesion of the matrix covered by normal nail-producing epithelium. Its connective tissue stroma is densely cellular and contains fine collagen fibres. The tumour projections fit into channels in the thickened nail substance that run along the whole length of the nail. After avulsion, the nail substance shows these channels lined with the upper third to half of normal matrix epithelium, exactly as seen on the nail's undersurface after nail avulsion. The exact nature of this lesion is not yet clear; however, human papillomavirus has not been demonstrated.

Subungual filamentous tumour

This small lesion is unique to the nail. Causing a whitish, greyish or brownish longitudinal streak usually not more than 1 mm in width running from the distal lunula to the free edge of the nail plate, the tumour consists of a rim of whorled keratin at the undersurface of the nail plate. It corresponds to a tiny digitiform epithelial projection in the distal matrix. Brownish discoloration is due to blood imbibition.

Ungual fibrokeratoma

Ungual fibrokeratomas may arise from the most proximal part of the matrix and remain in a supraungual position; arise from the medial portion of the matrix and remain intraungual (dissecting fibrokeratoma); or arise from the distal matrix or nail bed growing entirely under the nail. The lesion is histologically characterized by a dense core of longitudinally arranged collagen, almost complete lack of elastic fibres, oedema in its acral part, and hyperkeratosis of the tip which usually includes dried plasma globules that stain positive with PAS.

Koenen's ungual fibroma – seen in about half of patients with tuberous sclerosis – is histologically indistinguishable.

Matrix fibroma

Although the lesion has yet to be defined clinically, histological examination reveals a nodular tumour in the matrix consisting of dense, fine connective tissue fibres and many fibroblasts, which is thus almost identical to the stromal portion of onychomatricoma.

Myxoid pseudocyst

Myxoid pseudocyst is one of the most frequent degenerative lesions of the nail area. Most commonly located in the proximal nail fold, it starts with a myxomatoid degeneration of the connective tissue which at first contains thin strands of loose connective tissue and stellate fibroblasts. The mucin masses eventually enlarge and compress the marginal connective tissue to form a denser pseudocapsule. Neither immunohistochemistry nor electron microscopy has revealed a cyst lining of synovial cells even though the majority of pseudocysts later communicate with the adjacent distal interphalangeal joint.

Coccal nail-fold angiomatosis

A recently described reactive angiomatous lesion, coccal nail-fold angiomatosis, clinically and histologically resembles pyogenic granuloma. This lesion was observed in patients who had sustained severe trauma proximal to the digits involved, usually a fracture at the level of the wrist which had been treated with a splint; it was therefore also suggested to be a particular form of sympathetic reflex dystrophy. The tumours grow out from under the proximal nail fold, are erosive, and contain vascular proliferations in an oedematous stroma with many plasma cells and lymphocytes. The surface may be covered with cocci.

Glomus tumour

Even though glomus tumour is relatively rare, this hamartoma is well known for its characteristic symptoms. Histologically, a round, encapsulated organoid tumour is seen. It consists of an afferent arteriole, efferent vein and nerve supply. Vascular channels lined by a thin endothelium and surrounded by cuboidal cells lie in the loose, often myxomatoid stroma. Both myelinated and non-myelinated nerve fibres can be demonstrated.

Neurogenic tumours of the nail apparatus do not exhibit features different from tumours in other locations.

Subungual exostosis

Subungual exostosis is a relatively frequent lesion most commonly seen under the distal medial aspect of the hallux nail. It is a reactive growth probably due to repeated trauma. A broad-based growth of trabecular bone sits on the distal phalanx. It has a cap of fibrocartilage that may merge with hyaline cartilage, which forms new columns of bone by endochondral ossification. Both osteoblasts and osteoclasts may be seen.

Synovialoma

Giant cell tumour of the tendon sheath may involve the distal phalanx. It is a densely cellular tumour composed of histiocytes and fibroblasts with a variable proportion of giant cells that often resemble osteoclasts. Some foam cells and foci of siderophages are common.

Multicentric reticulohistiocytosis

Multiple small verrucous nodules at the margin of the proximal nail fold may be seen in multicentric reticulohistiocytosis. Histologically, there is a dense mass of histiocytic cells with a large proportion of multinucleated cells with a 'ground glass' appearance of the cytoplasm.

Melanocytic naevus of the nail organ

Naevi may be located at any site in or around the nail organ, and may pose considerable differential diagnostic problems when they cause longitudinal melanonychia. This sign may be due to a focus of functionally active melanocytes (as in ethnic pigmentation), to an accumulation of active melanocytes (as in the Laugier–Hunziker–Baran syndrome), or to a common lentigo, junctional melanocytic naevus, compound naevus or malignant melanoma.

Most naevi are of the junctional type. A few barely visible cells or large numbers of distinctly pigmented melanocytes may be seen singly or in clusters within the basal and suprabasal matrix epithelium. Mitoses are absent. A few melanophages may occur in the upper papillary. The nail plate contains intracellular fine melanin granules. Despite clinically obvious pigmentation, pigment visualization under the microscope often requires staining with the Fontana–Masson argentaffin reaction. Suprabasal location of melanocytes is common in the matrix and nail bed and must not be confused with melanoma.

Congenital and acquired compound naevi of the nail organ are similar to those of the skin.

Nail melanoma

Melanoma of the nail apparatus most commonly derives from the matrix, much less frequently from the nail bed or hyponychium. Matrix melanoma usually causes longitudinal melanonychia (see Chapter 5). Whether atypical melanocytic hyperplasia is already subungual *in situ* melanoma is not entirely clear. Large, atypical melanocytes in all layers of the matrix and nail bed epithelium, pycnotic melanocytes in the nail plate mirroring the pagetoid spread in the epithelium, and mitoses, are seen as proof of a malignant melanoma. Sometimes nail clippings reveal single intraungual pycnotic melanoma cells which retain their protein S-100 positivity.

Most subungual melanomas are of acrolentiginous type; however, those in the nail bed tend instead to be nodular melanomas. Even long-standing melanomas are often still very superficial. Invasive melanomas have therefore usually a decade-long history.

Epidermoid carcinoma

The term 'epidermoid carcinoma' denotes both ungual Bowen's disease and squamous cell carcinoma. Commonly originating from the lateral sulcus, Bowen's disease slowly spreads under and around the nail. Histologically, all changes typical of Bowen's disease of the skin are seen: loss of orderly architecture and polarity of basal cells, atypical nuclei, pathological mitoses, some giant cells, dyskeratoses, often vacuolization, and even clear cells. After decades the lesion develops into invasive squamous cell carcinoma, which, however, may also develop without prior bowenoid changes.

Malignant onycholemmal cyst is probably a particular form of Bowen's disease, as was seen in a case in which the cyst, after incomplete removal, rapidly showed the features of typical squamous cell carcinoma (author's unpublished observation).

FURTHER READING

Alessi E, Zorzi F, Gianotti R, Parafiori A (1994) Malignant proliferating onycholemmal cyst, *J Cut Pathol* **21**: 183–188.

Baran R, Goettmann S (1998) Distal digital keratoacanthoma: a report of 12 cases and review of the literature, *Br J Dermatol* **139**: 512–515.

Baran R, Kint A (1992) Onychomatrixoma. Filamentous tufted tumour in the matrix of a funnel-shaped nail: a new entity, *Br J Dermatol* **126**: 510–515.

Blessing K, Kernohan NM, Park KGM (1991) Subungual malignant melanoma. Clinicopathological features of 100 cases, *Histopathology* **19**: 425–429.

Davies MG (1995) Coccal nail fold angiomatosis, *Br J Dermatol* **132**: 162–163.

Haneke E (1983) Onycholemmal horn, *Dermatologica* **167**: 155–158.

Haneke E (1988) Operative Therapie der myxoiden Pseudocyste. In: *Gegenwärtiger Stand der operativen Dermatologie*, Haneke E, ed. (Berlin, Springer) pp. 221–227.

Haneke E (1991) Multiple subungual keratoacanthomas, *Zbl Haut GeschlKr* **159**: 337–338.

Haneke E (1991) Epidermoid carcinoma (Bowen's disease) of the nail simulating acquired fibrokeratoma, *Skin Cancer* **6**: 217–221.

Haneke E, Fränken J (1995) Onychomatricoma, *Dermatol Surg* **21**: 984–987.

Kint A, Baran R (1988) Histopathologic study of Koenen tumours, *J Am Acad Dermatol* **18**: 369–372.

Malvehy J, Palou J, Mascaró JM (1998) Painful subungual tumour in incontinentia pigmenti. Response to treatment with etretinate, *Br J Dermatol* **138**: 554–555.

11 Ultrasonography and magnetic resonance imaging of the perionychium

Jean-Luc Drapé, Sophie Goettmann, Alain Chevrot and Jacques Bittoun

Ultrasonography · **Magnetic resonance imaging** · **Conclusion** · **Further reading**

It may seem surprising to devote an entire chapter to imaging of the perionychium, as traditionally this structure has been difficult to investigate radiologically. However, high-frequency transducers now allow accurate ultrasonographic imaging of the finger tips. Magnetic resonance imaging (MRI) of the nail unit is also available, thanks to small dedicated surface coils. These new resources could modify the imaging strategy of ungual and subungual diseases.

The main indication for these new techniques is the investigation of nail tumours. Tumours of the perionychium may be difficult to diagnose because of this structure's anatomic peculiarities. Symptoms, growth, and above all the appearance of the tumours may be modified by the screen produced by the nail plate. Deep tumours that originate close to the nail root are covered by the posterior nail fold and may only be expressed by nail dystrophy. Thus, every suspect lesion of the nail unit should be investigated by radiography and biopsy. Complementary imaging should help in difficult cases by confirming and accurately locating the periungual mass.

Radiographs remain the essential means of imaging the nail unit. They are essential for study of the distal phalanx, but show very little of the soft tissues. The technique is adapted by use of high-resolution one-layer breast films or dedicated digital films. Posteroanterior and lateral views of the involved finger usually are sufficient. Oblique views may be necessary to highlight subtle erosions of the phalanx. Most nail dystrophies should benefit from radiography before surgical investigation. These radiographs can show abnormalities of the soft tissues, such as a thickening of the posterior nail fold with a mucoid cyst. Comparative lateral radiographs can highlight a difference in thickness of the nail bed when a subungual mass is present. Radiographs may depict soft-tissue calcifications as phleboliths of a haemangioma. Bone tumours may be suspected with pedicled ossifications of an exostosis, or mottled calcifications of a paraosteal chondroma. Enchondroma may expand the distal phalanx and be complicated by a pathologic fracture. Dense bone abnormalities may be secondary to an osteoid osteoma or to psoriatic arthropathy with periosteitis. When a mucoid cyst is suspected, a lateral view is suitable to highlight osteoarthritis of the distal interphalangeal phalanx with dorsal osteophytes impinging on the distal band of the extensor tendon. Erosion of the distal phalanx may be depicted in several diseases, as invasive subungual squamous carcinoma or keratoacanthomas, glomus tumours or epidermoid cysts.

ULTRASONOGRAPHY

Ultrasonography should be more widely used in imaging the nail unit. However, its dependence on operator skills and the moderate experience of radiologists in this anatomical region are limiting factors. High-frequency (7.5–20 MHz) probes dedicated to musculoskeletal or skin imaging are suitable. An interposition material is necessary for the study of the most superficial structures. The nail bed presents a somewhat homogeneous hypoechoic appearance, separating the high-intensity echoes of the dorsal cortex of the phalanx from those of the nail plate (Figure 11.1a). The nail plate may produce two parallel high-signal echoes. Imaging the matrix area is possible with 30 MHz B-mode, but is tricky because of the overlying echoes of the proximal and lateral nail folds. Furthermore, the axial slices are distorted by the convexity of the nail plate (Figure 11.1b). Ultrasonography was proposed as a way of detecting glomus tumours of the finger tips. Tumours less than 3 mm in diameter are hardly visible, but tumours located in the pulp are more accessible. Doppler imaging may reveal the vascular feature of this lesion in some cases (Figure 11.2). Ultrasonography is also appropriate for highlighting radiotransparent foreign bodies, such as splinters. A combined granulomatous reaction may be revealed with imaging.

Very high-resolution ultrasonographic studies are still restricted to the field of research,

beginning with skin imaging in 1979. Ultrasonography appeared as an effective and non-invasive method of measurement of the dermis thickness. Both A-mode and B-mode ultrasonographs dedicated to skin imaging have been developed as research and clinical tools, mainly for tumoral and inflammatory diseases. The role of M-mode, high-frequency Doppler imaging and three-dimensional investigations remains experimental. Probes of

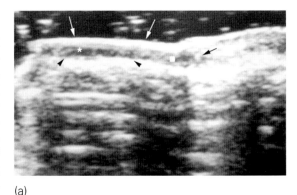

(a)

(b)

Figure 11.1
Ultrasonography of the nail unit. (a) Sagittal view. (b) Axial view. Nail plate (white arrows), nail bed (star), dorsal cortex of the phalanx (black arrowheads), nail root (black arrow), lateral nail fold (white arrowheads).

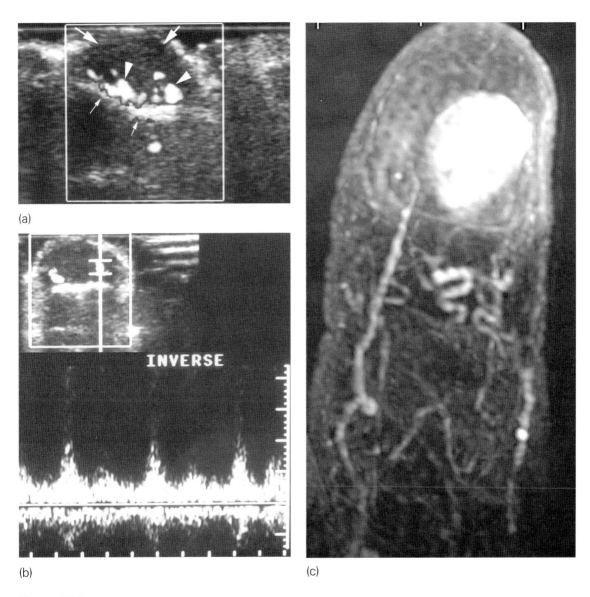

(a)

(b)

(c)

Figure 11.2
Subungual glomus tumour. (a) Color Doppler scan depicts a hypoechoic mass (large arrows) in the nail bed with vascular flow (arrowheads). Note bone erosion of the dorsal cortex of the distal phalanx (small arrows). (b) Pulsed Doppler with spectral analysis of the tumour. (c) Magnetic resonance angiography shows a highly vascularized mass beneath the nail plate.

20 MHz provide the best compromise between a high spatial resolution and sufficient depth. Probes of 50 MHz or more only allow imaging of the epidermis, with an axial resolution of about 37.5 μm and a lateral resolution of about 125 μm. Paradoxically, studies of the

nail unit are few. Finlay introduced ultrasonography for the assessment of the thickness of the nail plate with a 20 MHz A-mode probe. The distal conduction speeds (mean 2470 m/s) were well correlated with the measurements of the free edge of the nail plate with a micrometer. The distal reduction about 8.8% of the ultrasound transmission time compared with the proximal measurements should be due to a higher thickness and hydration of the nail plate at the level of the lunula. Jemec also studied the A-mode ultrasound structure of the nail plates of post-mortem thumbs *in situ* and after resection. The spatial resolution was about 75 µm with a 20 MHz probe. In contrast to Finlay, he noted compartments of different echo speeds, a superficial dry layer (ultrasound velocity of 3103 m/s) and a deep hydrated layer (ultrasound velocity of 2125 m/s). However, he could not differentiate the different layers of the nail bed. Hirai proposed 30 MHz B-mode ultrasonography to image nail matrix abnormalities in cases of nail plate deformities.

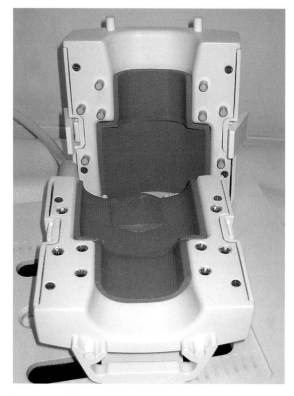

Figure 11.3
Phased array surface coil dedicated to wrist imaging.

MAGNETIC RESONANCE IMAGING

There have been a few reports of MRI investigations of subungual tumours, particularly glomus tumours. In practice the perionychium may be routinely imaged by MRI with the ability to obtain high spatial resolution images with small surface coils dedicated to wrist or finger (Figure 11.3). A voxel height close to 100 µm, about the thickness of the epithelial layer of the nail bed, is necessary. Nevertheless, unlike the skin, which is a superficial structure, the nail unit may require evaluation of the deep layers of the nail bed, or even of the pulp when the tumour extends under the lateral interosseous ligament. The thumbs and the great toes may be large, and it may be necessary to keep a sufficient

signal-to-noise ratio about 2 cm or more from the surface coil. When using a plane circular surface coil, the nail plate must be placed against the coil to offer the maximum signal close to the superficial layers of the nail unit. The hand is placed above the head in a supine or prone position with the coil fixed on the centre of the gantry. Full cooperation of the patient and efficient mechanical support with adhesive bandages are necessary. Some patients with painful shoulders (rotator cuff tears, multiple tendon calcifications) or frozen shoulder cannot maintain this position during the entire examination. For study of the toes, the position is more comfortable: the patient lies supine with the

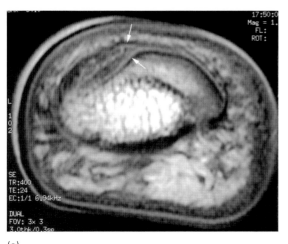

(a)

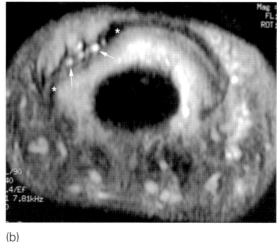

(b)

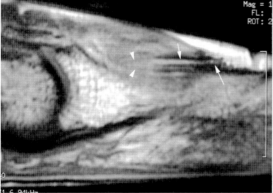

(c)

Figure 11.4
Onychomatricoma. (a) Axial T_1-weighted
magnetic resonance slice shows the tumour
seated between the dorsal and ventral nail
matrix (arrows). (b) Axial short-time inversion
recovery (STIR) slice depicts the high signal of
the filamentous expansions inside the nail plate
(star). (c) Sagittal T_1-weighted image shows the
tumour core (arrowheads) in the nail root and
its distal expansions (arrows).

feet in the gantry. In all cases perfect
immobility of the distal phalanx is necessary
to avoid movement artefacts, which are
particularly disturbing with high spatial
resolution. For this reason, children younger
than 6 years should not be examined in this
manner. Routine examination includes axial
T_1-weighted spin echo images (Figure 11.4a)
and axial fast short-time inversion recovery
(STIR) images (Figure 11.4b), completed with
sagittal T_1 or T_2 images (Figure 11.4c). The
slice thickness (usually 3 mm) remains large
compared with the size of the nail unit.
Three-dimensional gradient echo images are
acquired when 1 mm thick contiguous slices
are necessary (Figure 11.5). Coronal slices
are not acquired routinely. These slices are
disappointing, and are not adapted to the
spatial structure of the perionychium; they
are reserved for distal phalanx abnormalities
(Figure 11.6). Its different elements are
tangential to the frontal plane and therefore
exposed to the partial volume artefact.
Intravenous injection of 0.1 mmol/kg gadolinium is administered according to the
suspected pathological condition. Multiple
MR angiography sequences may be acquired
at arterial and venous phases (Figure 11.2c).

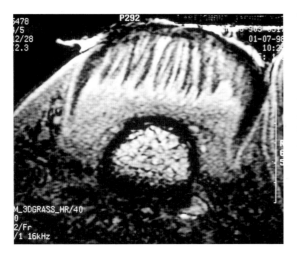

Figure 11.5
Onychomatricoma. Axial 1 mm thick three-dimensional gradient echo image highlights the filamentous expansions of the tumour.

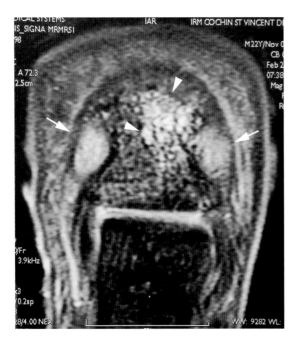

Figure 11.6
Osteoid osteoma of the distal phalanx. Axial post-gadolinium T_1-weighted coronal image depicts a bone oedema (arrowheads) of the tuft. Note the lateral Flint's ligaments (arrows).

Tumours of the perionychium

In the authors' institution the main indications for MRI are vascular tumours and mucoid cysts. Numerous other lesions are explored, such as epithelial tumours (warts, epidermoid cysts, onychomatricomas, keratoacanthomas), soft-tissue tumours (fibrokeratomas, fibromas, tenosynovial giant cell tumours), and osteochondral lesions (exostoses, chondromas, osteoid osteomas, chondrosarcomas). The accurate location of the tumour with MRI associated with its signal patterns is important for diagnosis.

Glomus tumours

Glomus tumours develop from the glomus bodies, which are particularly numerous in the dermis of the nail bed. High-resolution MRI is able to depict normal glomus bodies with T_2–weighted images and following injection of gadolinium. The classic triad associating pain, tenderness to pressure and cold sensitivity is evocative but infrequent. Imaging appears helpful to the diagnosis in 68% of cases. The mean diagnostic delay, varying from 4 to 7 years in published cases, should be shortened.

The signal behaviour of the glomus tumour depends on its histological composition. These tumours are the result of hyperplasia of one or several elements of the glomus bodies, and they may be considered to be hamartomas. In 1924, Masson described a number of histological variants. These are not routinely mentioned in pathology reports, as they have no prognostic significance; however, knowledge of them is important in evaluating the tumour signal:

1   Vascular tumours are composed of numerous vascular lumens. Enhancement is high after injection of gadolinium, and the signal is high on T_2-weighted images. Angiographic MRI shows an early enhancement at the arterial phase, increasing at the delayed venous acquisition (Figure 11.7).

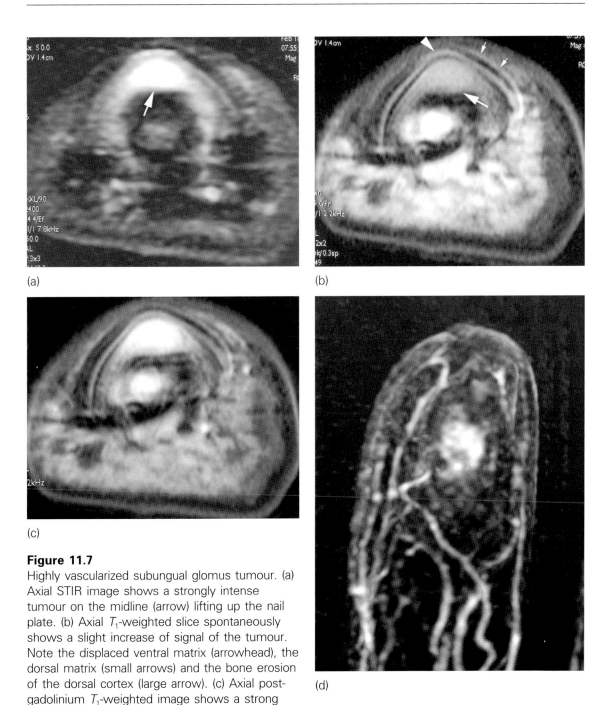

Figure 11.7
Highly vascularized subungual glomus tumour. (a) Axial STIR image shows a strongly intense tumour on the midline (arrow) lifting up the nail plate. (b) Axial T_1-weighted slice spontaneously shows a slight increase of signal of the tumour. Note the displaced ventral matrix (arrowhead), the dorsal matrix (small arrows) and the bone erosion of the dorsal cortex (large arrow). (c) Axial post-gadolinium T_1-weighted image shows a strong and homogeneous enhancement of the glomus tumour. (d) Magnetic resonance angiography confirms the high degree of vascularization of the tumour on the delayed sequence.

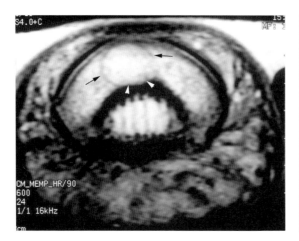

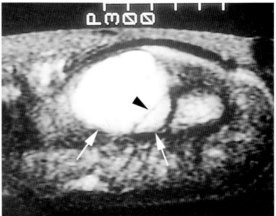

Figure 11.8
Solid form of glomus tumour. Axial post-gadolinium T_1-weighted image shows a tumour with a signal equal to the signal of the nail bed. The tumour is highlighted by its peripheral low-signal pseudocapsule (arrows) and the bone erosion (arrowheads).

Figure 11.9
Mucoid type of glomus tumour. Sagittal T_2-weighted image depicts a tumour with a high signal (arrows) and an internal septum (arrowhead).

2   Cellular or solid tumours mainly present a proliferation of epithelioid cells (glomus cells) and a relative paucity of vascular lumens. This type of tumour is difficult to detect with MRI. Its signal is close to that of the normal dermis of the nail bed on all sequences. Injection of gadolinium, even with MR angiography, is of little use. Thin, three-dimensional contiguous gradient echo slices are the most helpful by depicting a peripheral capsule or a slight bone erosion on the dorsal aspect of the phalanx (Figure 11.8).

3   Mucoid tumours, with mucoid degeneration of the stroma, present a faint enhancement but have a very high signal on T_2–weighted images due to the large amount of water in the stroma (Figure 11.9).

Numerous tumours are a combination of these three elementary types (Figure 11.10). Most often the tumour limits are well defined

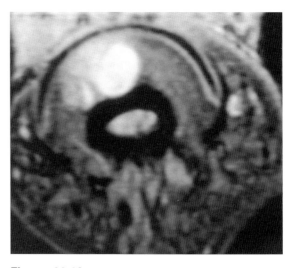

Figure 11.10
Mixed glomus tumour. Axial post-gadolinium three-dimensional gradient echo image shows heterogeneous enhancement of the tumour.

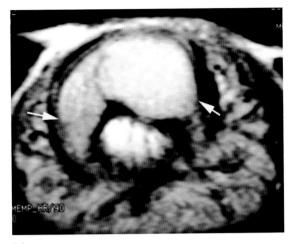

(a)

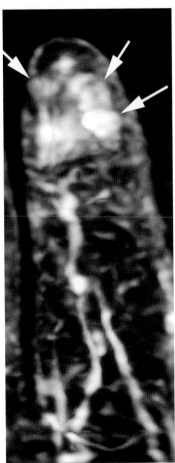

(b)

Figure 11.11
Multiple glomus tumours. (a) Axial post-gadolinium T_1-weighted slice depicts two tumours in the nail bed on both sides of the midline (arrows) with bone erosions. (b) Magnetic resonance angiography shows multiple nodular enhancement in the nail bed (arrows).

with a peripheral pseudocapsule (see Figure 11.8). This capsule is a reactional response of the surrounding connective tissue; it presents a low signal on all sequences, but is more visible on T_2-weighted images or three-dimensional gradient echo images. In some cases the tumour limits are ill defined, and injection of gadolinium – particularly with MR angiography – may depict small foci of tumour extending into the nearby nail bed (Figure 11.11). Often in these cases, adhesions with the nail bed are noted during surgery. Local invasion of the capsule is debated; it has been reported on histological examinations in less than 2% of cases. It is certain that the risk of recurrence is high if some tumoral tissue is left *in situ* during surgery of these ill-defined lesions. The reported recurrence rate varies from 12% to 24%. Magnetic resonance imaging appears to be particularly helpful in cases of recurrent pain after surgery (Figure 11.12). Magnetic resonance angiography also is able to depict multiple glomus tumours in the hand or in the same finger tip. In these cases, MRI is essential for planning the surgical approach (Figure 11.13).

In most cases the tumour is located in the subungual area, in the supporting tissue of the nail bed or the matrix. These locations are the most difficult to depict with ultrasonography when the tumour is smaller than 3 mm. Usually the lesion is deep, close to the periosteum of the underlying phalanx. Often a cortical bone erosion is depicted on the axial slices although it was occult on radiographs. These axial slices are essential to distinguish the tumours on the median line from those of the lateral part of the nail bed, which sometimes extend into the pulp via the rima ungualum. The surgical approach is planned according to the size and location of the tumour. Lateral tumours may be excised by a lateral approach while the median type may require a transungual approach. Sagittal slices are essential to determine the relations between the tumour and the nail matrix. Unusually, the lesions may

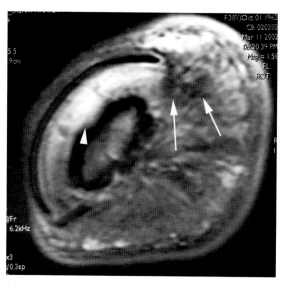

(a)

Figure 11.12

Postoperative recurrent glomus tumour. (a) Axial post-gadolinium T_1-weighted image faintly shows a recurrent tumour in the nail bed with a bone erosion (arrowhead). Note the artefacts (arrows) of the previous surgery on the lateral nail fold. (b) Magnetic resonance angiography highlights the enhancement of the glomus tumour. Note the dark postoperative artefact (arrow) close to the tumour.

be located in the pulp or the posterior nail fold; in such cases, the contrast between healthy tissue and tumour is completely different because of the fatty tissue of the hypodermis surrounding the tumour. The low-signal tumour is spontaneously visible on T_1-weighted images, surrounded by the high signal of fat. The tumour enhancement after injection of gadolinium is only visible with associated fat suppression (Figure 11.14).

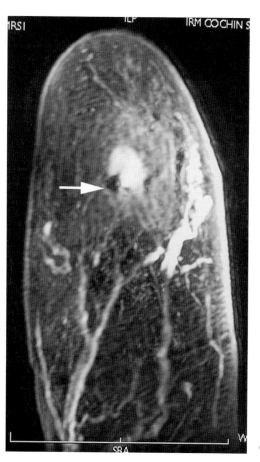

(b)

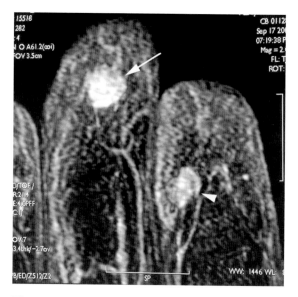

Figure 11.13

Multiple glomus tumours involving the third (arrow) and fourth (arrowhead) finger tips, seen on MR angiography.

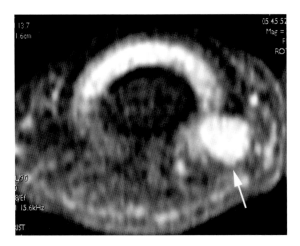

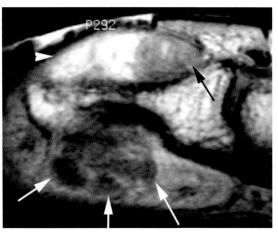

Figure 11.14
Glomus tumour seated in the pulp and the rima ungualum. Axial fat-suppressed post-gadolinium T_1-weighted image depicts the tumour enhancement (arrow) surrounded by the low signal of fat.

Figure 11.15
Vascular malformation of the finger tip. Sagittal post-gadolinium T_1-weighted image depicts a thickened nail bed invaded by a thrombosed (black arrow) and an enhanced (arrowhead) vascular malformation. Note the extension towards the pulp with numerous flow void artefacts (white arrows) due to high blood velocity.

Glomus tumours are easily distinguished from other vascular lesions, such as venous haemangiomas and arteriovenous malformations, by their characteristic blood flow artefacts and vascular pedicles.

Other vascular tumours

Vascular tumours that involve the perionychium are mostly benign, except for Kaposi's sarcoma. The histological types are numerous, from the exceptional haemangioma of the nail bed to the capillary malformations present from birth. Radiographs can depict a mass in the soft tissues, phleboliths, and even a bone erosion with venous and arteriovenous malformations, or an epithelioid haemangiendothelioma. The bone may be primarily involved by a haemangioma (linear striations parallel to the shaft of the phalanx) or an aneurysmal bone cyst (expansive osteolytic lesion of the phalanx). It is not possible to differentiate all these types of vascular lesions by MRI, but discrimination is improved with MR angiography. The vascular nature often is obvious with high-flow malformations (flow void artefacts) and low-flow lesions (very bright signal on T_2-weighted images) (Figure 11.15). Manetic resonance imaging assesses the extension of the lesion into the soft tissues and MR angiography the angioarchitecture of the malformation and its relations with the digital collateral arteries and the venous plexus.

Mucoid cysts

Complementary imaging of mucoid cysts may seem irrelevant because the clinical diagnosis is easy; most of the cysts originate from the accessible posterior nail fold. However, the high

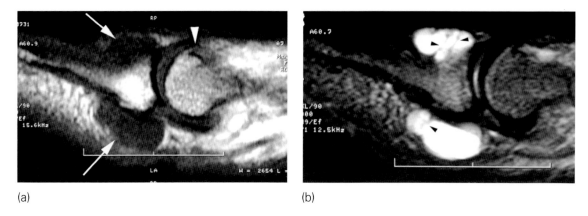

(a)   (b)

Figure 11.16
Mucoid cyst of the proximal nail fold and the pulp (arrows). (a) Sagittal T_1-weighted image; note the dorsal osteophyte of the phalangeal head (arrowhead). (b) Sagittal T_2-weighted image. Note the intracystic septa (arrowheads).

recurrence rate despite numerous treatment possibilities may increase the interest in accurate preoperative imaging. High-resolution MRI can accurately analyse the relations between the cyst and the distal interphalangeal joint. Most of the cysts are solitary and located on the proximal nail fold. Their appearance is specific: thin, regular walls, low signal on T_1-weighted images and very high signal on T_2-weighted images. Intracystic septa are best seen on T_2-weighted images in 39% of cases (Figure 11.16). Injection of gadolinium shows early faint peripheral enhancement and with time the enhancement moves toward the centre of the cyst. This diffusion of contrast media may be compared to the intra-articular diffusion of gadolinium at the level of the knee through the synovium after intravenous injection of gadolinium. However, a true synovial membrane has not been found in digital cysts, apart from a possible peduncle. Magnetic resonance imaging is able to highlight satellite cysts or sagging multiloculated cysts (Figure 11.17). These latter forms may be difficult to detect clinically, unless the typical signs of swelling and discharge of a thick fluid from the proximal nail fold are found. In these infrequent

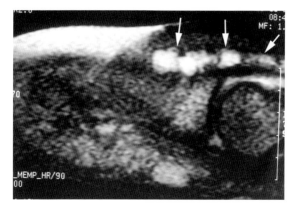

Figure 11.17
Sagging multilocated mucoid cyst (arrowed) of the proximal nail fold – sagittal T_2-weighted image.

forms (22%) it was not possible to detect a connection with the distal interphalangeal joint. These cysts may develop independently from the underlying joint and result from increased production of hyaluronic acid due to the metaplasia of fibroblasts. This process may be compared to the cutaneous myxomas with a focal storage of mucoid material in the dermis.

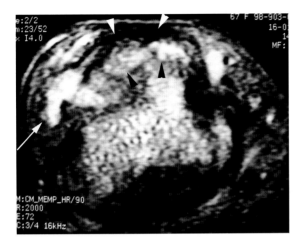

Figure 11.18
Mucoid cyst of the proximal nail fold – axial T_2-weighted image. A dorsal osteophyte (black arrowheads) lifts up the terminal band of the extensor tendon (white arrowheads). Note the underlying peduncle of the mucoid cyst (arrow).

A peduncle connecting the cyst and the distal interphalangeal joint is visible by MRI in most cases. In all these cases the peduncle is lateral, beneath the insertion of the extensor digitorum tendon on the base of the distal phalanx (Figure 11.18). If surgical treatment is chosen, the peduncle must be detected and tied up or removed to avoid frequent recurrences. The peroperative injection of methyl blue mixed with hydrogen peroxide into the palmar aspect of the distal interphalangeal joint to colour this peduncle has been proposed to aid in its identification, but this is not always easy to do.

Mucoid cysts extend into the nail bed in 30% of cases, a location that has been neglected by research. Symptoms may lead to misdiagnosis of glomus tumour when the cyst is painful. High-resolution MRI is able to detect this type of cyst. When the cyst is large, erosion of the cortex of the underlying phalanx may occur in the confined space of the nail bed. The cyst is in the dermis beneath the nail matrix, close to the distal interphalangeal joint

(Figure 11.19). Matrix compression may induce a fissure of the nail plate with a claw deformity. Most often, the cyst is bilobar, with a component in the proximal nail fold (more rarely in the pulp) associated with the nail bed component. The submatrical extension may be

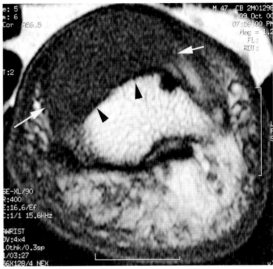

(a)

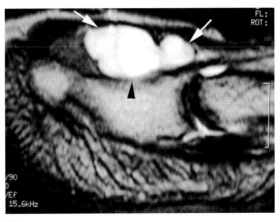

(b)

Figure 11.19
Subungual mucoid cyst (arrows). (a) Axial T_1-weighted image. (b) Sagittal T_2-weighted image. Note bone erosion (arrowhead).

clinically occult and responsible for recurrence. Detection of a peduncle is crucial, because its resection may be enough to collapse the cyst and avoid direct access to the matrix.

Epithelial tumours

Epidermoid cysts of the distal phalanx are rare, usually secondary to trauma with implantation of epidermis into subcutaneous tissue or even into bone. An old trauma often goes unnoticed. The cyst may develop on a scar after surgery. The phalanx progressively expands and clubbing becomes obvious. The pain is of late onset, sometimes on the occasion of a pathological fracture. Histological investigation shows an epidermoid cyst filled with orthokeratin and lined with a thin layer of epidermis. Radiographs depict a round, accurately rimmed erosion of the distal phalanx without septa or peripheral sclerosis. In early stages the bone erosion is absent or subtle and is occult on radiographs. Magnetic resonance imaging shows a regular mass with slight heterogeneous content and intermediate signal on T_1-weighted and T_2-weighted images; heterogeneous enhancement is noted after injection of gadolinium (Figure 11.20). A thin, regular rim with a high signal identical to that of normal epidermis is due to the peripheral epidermal layer. Bone erosions, even subtle, are highly visible on axial images. The area of an old penetrating injury may be marked by dark artefacts on gradient-echo images.

Keratoacanthoma is a rare, benign, but rapidly growing tumour located in the most distal part of the nail bed. The lesion may start as a small, painful keratotic nodule beneath the free edge of the nail plate. Magnetic resonance imaging shows a dome-shaped nodule with a homogeneous signal (intermediate on T_1, hyperechoic on T_2) and strong enhancement. A central area of low signal may indicate a central plug of horny material filling

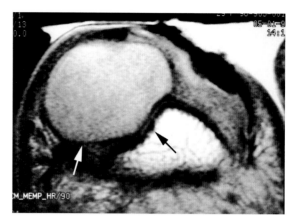

Figure 11.20
Epidermoid cyst – axial T_1-weighted image. The cyst appears spontaneously with a slight high signal. Bone erosion is arrowed.

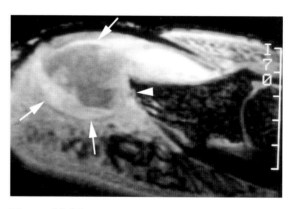

Figure 11.21
Keratoacanthoma. Sagittal post-gadolinium T_1-weighted image showing strong peripheral enhancement (arrow) and acro-osteolysis (arrowhead).

the crater, but this is inconstant. The limits may be ill defined owing to oedema in the surrounding tissues. Magnetic resonance images show a deep infiltrating lesion and detect more accurately than radiographs a frequent bone erosion (Figure 11.21).

Onychomatricomas must be suspected from clinical signs, with a filamentous tufted tumour in the matrix of a funnel-shaped nail. Histologically there is epithelial proliferation of the matrix or surrounding epidermis. The lobules are delimited by normal basal cells and are composed of keratinocytes identical to those of the matrix. After removal of these parakeratotic cells, an invagination remains resembling the infundibulum of a hair follicle. Sagittal MRI is essential to highlight the tumoral core in the matrical area and the invagination of the lesion into the funnel-shaped nail plate (see Figure 11.4). The centre shows a low signal on all sequences, with a peripheral rim with a signal identical to that of normal epidermis. The distal part with the filamentous extensions presents a higher signal on T_2-weighted images due to a mucoid stroma (see Figure 11.5). Axial slices accurately show the holes in the substance of the nail plate, filled with the filamentous extensions.

CONCLUSION

Imaging of the nail unit tends to be limited to X-rays. However, ultrasonography has a valuable role in detecting tumours or foreign bodies in soft tissues. Recent advances in high-resolution MRI allow further investigation of the nail unit. Accurate assessment of the extension of subungual tumours, such as glomus tumours, is now possible preoperatively.

FURTHER READING

Alexander H, Miller DL (1979) Determining skin thickness with pulsed ultrasound, *J Invest Dermatol* **72**: 17–19.

Baran R, Kechijian P (1989) Longitudinal melanonychia: diagnosis and management, *J Am Acad Dermatol* **21**: 1165–1175.

Baran R, Klint A (1992) Onychomatrixoma, *Br J Dermatol* **126**: 510–515.

Bittoun J, Leroy-Willig A, Idy I et al (1987) Relation entre rapport signal-sur-bruit et paramètres d'acquisition en IRM pour un contraste donné, *Ann Radiol* **30**: 5–13.

Camirand P, Rowe WF (1970) Subungual glomus tumour. Radiological manifestations, *Arch Dermatol* **102**: 677–679.

Carroll RE, Berman AT (1972) Glomus tumors of the hand: review of the literature and report of 28 cases, *J Bone Joint Surg* **54A**: 691–703.

Dailiana ZH, Drapé JL, Le Viet D (1999) A glomus tumour with four recurrences, *J Hand Surg* **24B**: 131–132.

Davis TS, Graham WP, Blomain EW (1986) A ten-year experience with glomus tumors, *Ann Plast Surg* **6**: 297–299.

Drapé JL, Thelen P, Gay-Depassier P et al (1993) Intraarticular diffusion of Gd-DPTA after intravenous injection in the knee: MR imaging evaluation, *Radiology* **188**: 227–234.

Drapé JL, Idy-Peretti I, Goettmann S et al (1995) MR imaging of subungual glomus tumors, *Radiology* **195**: 507–515.

Drapé JL, Idy-Peretti I, Goettmann S et al (1996) MR imaging of digital mucoid cysts, *Radiology* **200**: 531–536.

Drewers J, Günther D, Nolden HH (1985) Intraossäre epidermiszysten der finger und zehen, *Akt Chir* **20**: 171.

El-Gammal S, Hoffmann K, Auer T et al. (1991) A 50-MHz high-resolution ultrasound imaging system for dermatology. In: *Ultrasound in Dermatology*, eds Altemeyer P, El-Gammal S, Hoffmann K (Berlin, Springer) pp. 41–54.

Finlay AY, Moseley H, Duggan TC (1987) Ultrasound transmission time: an in vivo guide to nail thickness, *Br J Dermatol* **117**: 765–770.

Finlay AY, Western B, Edwards C (1990) Ultrasound velocity in human finger nail and effects of hydratation: validation of in vivo nail thickness measurement techniques, *Br J Dermatol* **123**: 365–373.

Fornage BD (1988) Glomus tumours in the fingers: diagnosis with ultrasound, *Radiology* **167**: 183–185.

Gandon F, Legaillard P, Brueton R *et al* (1992) Forty-eight glomus tumors of the hand: retrospective study and four-year follow-up, *Ann Hand Surg* **11**: 401–405.

Goldman L (1962) Transillumination of the fingertip as aid in examination of the nail changes, *Arch Dermatol Chicago* **85**: 644.

Hirai T, Fumiiri M (1995) Ultrasonic observation of the nail matrix, *Dermatol Surg* **21**: 158–161.

Hou SM, Shih TTF, Lin MC (1993) Magnetic resonance imaging of an obscure glomus tumour in the fingertip, *J Hand Surg* **18B**: 482–483.

Jablon M, Horowitz A, Bernstein DA (1990) Magnetic resonance imaging of a glomus tumor of the finger tip, *J Hand Surg* **15A**: 507–509.

Jemec GBE, Serup J (1989) Ultrasound structure of the nail plate, *Arch Dermatol* **125**: 643–646.

Keeney GL, Banks PM, Linscheild RL (1988) Subungual keratoacanthoma. Report of a case and review of the literature, *Arch Dermatol* **124**: 1074–1076.

Kneeland JB, Middelton WD, Matloub HS *et al* (1987) High resolution MR imaging of glomus tumor, *J Comput Assist Tomogr* **11**: 351–352.

Kohout E, Stout AP (1961) The glomus tumor in children, *Cancer* **14**: 555–556.

Lumpkin LR, Rosen T, Tschen JA (1984) Subungual squamous cell carcinoma, *J Am Acad Dermatol* **11**: 735–738.

Masson P (1924) Le glomus neuromyo-artériel des régions tactiles et ses tumeurs, *Lyon Chir* **21**: 256–280.

Mathis WH, Schulz MD (1948) Roentgen diagnosis of glomus tumours, *Radiology* **51**: 71–76.

Matloub HS, Muoneke VN, Prevel CD *et al* (1992) Glomus tumor imaging: use of MRI for localization of occult lesions, *J Hand Surg* **17A**: 472–475.

Newmeyer WL, Kilgore ES, Graham WP (1974) Mucous cyst: the dorsal distal interphalangeal joint ganglion, *Plast Reconstr Surg* **53**: 313–315.

Ogino T, Ohnishi N (1993) Ultrasonography of a subungual glomus tumour, *J Hand Surg* **18B**: 746–747.

Rettig AC, Strickland JW (1977) Glomus tumors of the digits, *J Hand Surg* **2A**: 261–265.

Schneider LH, Bachow TB (1991) Magnetic resonance imaging of glomus tumor, *Orthop Rev* **20**: 255–256.

Serup J (1991) Ten year's experience with high-frequency ultrasound examination of the skin: development and refinement of technique and equipment. In: *Ultrasound in Dermatology*, eds Altmeyer P, El-Gammal S, Hoffmann K (Berlin, Springer) pp. 41–54.

Tan CY, Marks R, Payne P (1981) Comparison of xeroradiographic and ultrasound detection of corticosteroid induced dermal thinning, *J Invest Dermatol* **76**: 126–128.

Varian J, Cleak DK (1980) Glomus tumors in the hand, *Hand* **12**: 293–299.

12 Dermoscopy of nail pigmentation

Luc Thomas and Sandra Ronger

Dermoscopy equipment · **Semiological patterns** · **Diagnosis** · **Further reading**

Diagnosis of melanonychia striata is one of the most difficult aspects of clinical dermatology. Melanoma is feared in most situations; however, melanoma of the nail apparatus is rare (about 1% of all cutaneous melanomas). The clinical presentation of early nail apparatus melanoma – longitudinal pigmentation – is shared by many other clinical processes with much more favourable outcomes, such as nail apparatus naevus or lentigo, drug-induced pigmentation, subungual haemorrhage and ethnic-type nail pigmentation. The 'gold standard' of diagnosis remains the pathological examination of the nail matrix biopsy, but the biopsy procedure is usually painful and often results in nail dystrophy.

Clinical criteria have been defined in an attempt to discriminate between suspect lesions that should undergo nail apparatus biopsy and less suspect ones that can just be followed-up. Suspicious signs are the occurrence of the pigmentation during adulthood, monodactlylic location of the pigmentation, heterogeneity of the pigmentation, and its progressive enlargement. Lesions more likely to be benign are those present since childhood, multiple lesions on several fingers and toes, and stable and homogeneously coloured lesions.

Dermoscopy provides additional evidence on which to base the decision to proceed with nail apparatus biopsy. This chapter describes the different patterns observed on epiluminescence microscopy and their relevance in the differential diagnosis of a nail pigmentation. Dermoscopy can also be used in the diagnosis of other nail conditions, for example the observation of vascular abnormalities associated with scleroderma or systemic lupus erythematosus.

DERMOSCOPY EQUIPMENT

Dermoscopy on nails can be performed using any type of hand-held dermoscope. After trying different compounds the authors have adopted a clear antiseptic gel (Purell, Gojo Industries Inc., Akron, Ohio, USA) for immersion, but ultrasonography gel may also be used provided it is not coloured. All the pictures in this chapter have been taken with a standard dermoscopic camera (Heine Dermaphot, Herrshing, Germany).

SEMIOLOGICAL PATTERNS

On the basis of a prospective study of 148 cases of linear nail pigmentation we have identified seven different semiological patterns:

1 Blood spots: these spots are characterized by a homogeneous colour. Recently formed lesions are purple and round; they turn brown and develop a more linear pattern with time. In older lesions the proximal edge of the spot remains sharply demarcated with an ovoid or polycyclic proximal border, while the distal edge appears elongated with creation of a somewhat filamentous pattern (see Figures 12.11, 12.12).

2 Brown background: in this pattern, usually associated with regular or irregular lines, the background of the area corresponding to the pigmented band appears homogeneously brown (Figures 12.1–12.6).

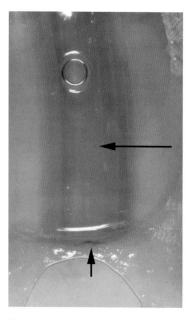

Figure 12.1
Nail apparatus melanoma ALM-type, Clark's level II, 0.2 mm thickness in a finger nail. Dermoscopy shows a brown background with irregularly pigmented lines (long arrow). A faint pigmentation of the cuticle is only visible on epiluminescence microscopy (micro-Hutchinson's sign) (short arrow). (Figures 12.1–12.12 are reproduced with kind permission of Josep Malvehy, editor of the *Atlas of Dermoscopy*.)

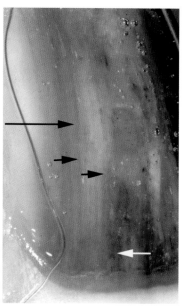

Figure 12.2
Nail apparatus melanoma, ALM-type, Clark's level III, 0.6 mm thickness in a thumb nail. Dermoscopy shows a brown background (long black arrow) and brown longitudinal bands with irregular spacing, pigmention and thickness (short black arrows). Note that blood spots are present (white arrow). Some areas of parallel disruption of the bands are also visible.

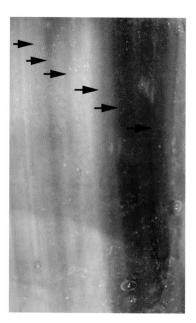

Figure 12.3
Nail apparatus melanoma, ALM-type, Clark's level III, 0.65 mm thickness in the great toe nail. Dermoscopy shows a brown background and longitudinal bands of irregular spacing, pigmentation and thickness (arrows).

3 Brown, longitudinal parallel lines with regular coloration, spacing and thickness and absence of parallelism disruption: this pattern is usually associated with a brown background and the lines appear superimposed on it. The colouration of the lines varies between lesions, from light brown to black, but the shade is consistent within each lesion. The spacing between bands is regular, and the thickness of the bands is also similar throughout the whole lesion (Figures 12.4–12.6).

4 Longitudinal, brown to black lines with irregular thickness, spacing or coloration and parallelism disruption: this pattern is also usually associated with a brown background, but the superimposed lines are heterogeneous with noticeable variegation

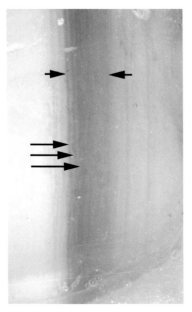

Figure 12.4
Nail apparatus melanocytic naevus in an adult's finger nail. Dermoscopy shows a brown background (between the two short arrows) and longitudinal bands with regular spacing, pigmentation and thickness (long arrows).

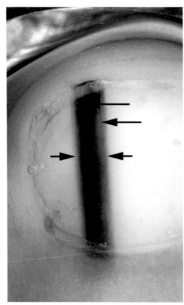

Figure 12.5
Nail apparatus melanocytic naevus in a child's finger nail. Dermoscopy shows a brown background (between the two short arrows) and longitudinal bands with regular spacing, pigmentation and thickness (long arrows). Note that the overall pigmentation is much darker than in Figure 12.4.

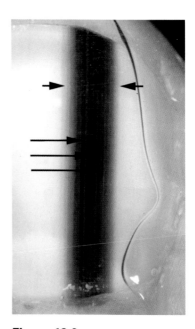

Figure 12.6
Nail apparatus melanocytic naevus in an adult's finger nail. Dermoscopy shows a brown background (between the two short arrows) and longitudinal bands with regular spacing, pigmentation and thickness (long arrows).

in their coloration, spacing and thickness. This heterogeneity of the bands is also asymmetrically disposed in the area of the clinically visible pigmented band. In some areas the bands have a curved shape or abruptly interrupt their pigmentation, disrupting the parallelism of the bands (see Figures 12.2 and 12.3).

5 Homogeneous greyish lines with grey pigmentation of the background: a greyish background with superimposed thin grey lines characterizes this pattern (see Figures 12.7–12.10).

6 Micro-Hutchinson's sign: clinically, Hutchinson's sign is the pigmentation of the cuticle in the area corresponding to the pigmented nail band; it suggests the presence of melanoma yet its specificity is not absolute. Dermoscopically the micro-Hutchinson sign can be defined as a pigmentation of the cuticle, invisible to the naked eye and only observable with epiluminescent skin surface examination. Other authors have described prominent pigmentation of periungual tissue and found that irregular pattern of distribution of the pigment on dermoscopy was strongly indicative of melanoma (see Figure 12.1).

7 Microscopic longitudinal grooves: these grooves appear as microscopic superficial fractures of the nail plate. They are not always superimposed on the pigmented band and can be observed in several nail conditions. In our opinion these grooves are non-specific and do not indicate any diagnosis (see Figure 12.8).

DIAGNOSIS

Nail apparatus naevus

Nail apparatus pigmented naevus is characterized dermoscopically by the presence of a

brown background and regularly spaced, thick and pigmented longitudinal lines. The colour of the background and of the bands varies from light brown to almost black from one lesion to another, but overall pigmentation is fairly consistent within any given lesion. The darkness of the pigmentation should not be regarded as particularly suspicious, but darker lesions may be difficult to analyse by epiluminescence microscopy (Figures 12.4–12.6).

Nail apparatus melanoma

In the authors' experience ungual melanoma is dermoscopically characterized by a brown background and the presence of irregular lines. These lines are different in colour from one another, and their thickness varies dramatically from one to another, as does the inter-band spacing. In some areas the bands abruptly stop and in other areas their parallelism is disrupted (Figures 12.2, 12.3).

Micro-Hutchinson's sign is rare and we have observed this feature in melanoma only. However, it is known from previous clinical studies that pigmentation of the cuticle is not completely specific to melanoma. In more advanced cases the pigmentation of periungual tissue appears irregular on dermoscopy (Figure 12.1).

Blood spots may be found in melanoma, therefore their presence should not mislead the clinician to a diagnosis of subungual haemorrhage.

Nail apparatus lentigo

Nail apparatus lentigo is in our experience a common condition. It is dermoscopically characterized by a greyish background with thin, superimposed grey lines. This pattern is shared with drug-induced nail pigmentation and ethnic nail pigmentation. Ungual lentigos in lentiginoses, such as Laugier–Hunziker–Baran disease, have the same dermoscopic appearance (Figures 12.7, 12.8).

Drug-induced nail pigmentation

Drug-induced pigmentation of the nail plate is usually easy to diagnose from the medical history of the patient, but some cases may be more difficult. Dermoscopic examination reveals a greyish band with thin grey lines, resembling lentigo (Figure 12.9).

Ethnic nail pigmentation

Ethnic nail pigmentation is usually easy to recognize by its familial inheritance and the polydactylic distribution of the bands. When observed with epiluminescence microscopy the bands have a fairly homogeneous grey background and thin grey lines comparable with those observed in lentigo (Figure 12.10).

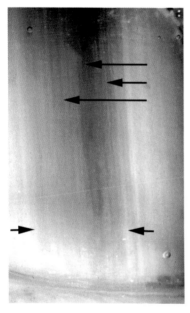 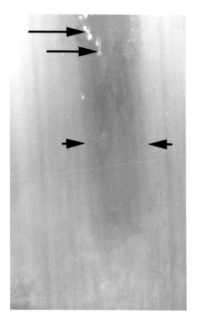 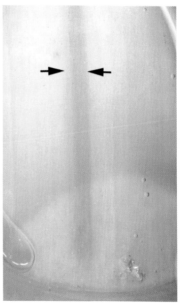

Figure 12.7
Ungual lentigo in an adult's finger nail. Dermoscopy reveals a relatively homogeneous greyish background (between the two short arrows) and superimposed thin grey lines (long arrows).

Figure 12.8
Ungual lentigo in an adult's toe nail. Dermoscopy shows a broad grey band with faint, thin grey lines (between the two short arrows). Note the presence of aspecific longitudinal microscopic grooves (long arrows).

Figure 12.9
Hydroxyurea-induced pigmentation of an adult's finger nail. The dermoscopic pattern is similar to that of lentigo, with a greyish background and thin grey lines (between the two short arrows).

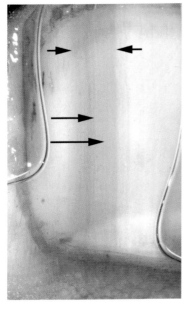

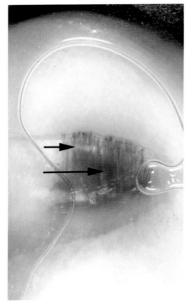

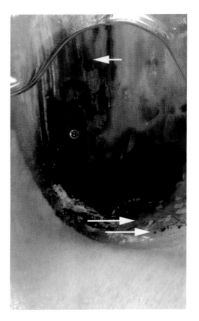

Figure 12.10
Ethnic-type pigmentation of a toe nail plate in an adult of Hispanic descent. Dermoscopy shows a greyish background (between the two short arrows) and thin superimposed grey lines (long arrows).

Figure 12.11
Subungual haemorrhage in a child's toe nail (old lesion). Note the elongated, parallel linear pattern of the distal edge of the pigmentation (short arrow) and the purple–brown proximal blood spot (long arrow).

Figure 12.12
Subungual haemorrhage in an adult's great toe nail (recent lesion). The pigmentation is characteristically purple with an elongated parallel linear pattern at the distal edge (short arrow) and a well-demarcated, rounded proximal edge with characteristic features of blood spots (long arrows).

Subungual haemorrhage

Subungual haemorrhages often look alarming, especially when band-shaped. Dermoscopy provides powerful arguments for this diagnosis in the presence of blood spots (Figures 12.11, 12.12). However, as described above, blood spots are not uncommon in melanoma and diagnosis of subungual haemorrhage should only be made in the absence of brown lines. This negative criterion is of tremendous importance.

FURTHER READING

Banfield CC, Dawber RP (1996) Nail apparatus melanoma, *J Am Acad Dermatol* **34**: 322.

Banfield CC, Redburn JC, Dawber RP (1998) The incidence and prognosis of nail apparatus melanoma. A retrospective study of 105 patients in four English regions, *Br J Dermatol* **139**: 276–279.

Baran R (1978) Pigmentations of the nails (chromonychia). *J Dermatol Surg Oncol* **4**: 250–254.

Baran R, Kechijian P (1989) Longitudinal melanonychia (melanonychia striata): diagnosis and management, *J Am Acad Dermatol* **21**: 1165–1175.

Causeret A, Skowron F, Viallard A, Balme B, Thomas L (2002) Subungueal blue naevus, *J Am Acad Dermatol* (in press).

Fernando SS, Lauer CS (1987) The diagnostic dilemma of subungual melanoma, *Med J Aust* **146**: 325.

Fleegler EJ (1992) A surgical approach to melanonychia striata, *J Dermatol Surg Oncol* **18**: 708–714.

Fountain JA (1990) Recognition of subungual hematoma as an imitator of subungual melanoma, *J Am Acad Dermatol* **23**: 773–774.

Goettmann-Bonvallot S, Andre J, Belaich S (1999) Longitudinal melanonychia in children: a clinical and histopathologic study of 40 cases, *J Am Acad Dermatol* **41**: 17–22.

Haneke E (1991) [Laugier–Hunziker–Baran syndrome.] *Hautarzt* **42**: 512–515.

Haneke E, Baran R (2001) Longitudinal melanonychia, *Dermatol Surg* **27**: 580–584.

Johr RH, Izakovic J (2001) Dermatoscopy/ELM for the evaluation of nail-apparatus pigmentation, *Dermatol Surg* **27**: 315–322.

Kawabata Y, Ohara K, Hino H, Tamaki K (2001) Two kinds of Hutchinson's sign, benign and malignant, *J Am Acad Dermatol* **44**: 305–307.

Kikuchi I, Inoue S, Sakaguchi E, Ono T (1993) Regressing nevoid nail melanosis in childhood, *Dermatology* **186**: 88–93.

Norton LA (1980) Nail disorders. A review, *J Am Acad Dermatol* **2**: 451–467.

Rich P (1992) Nail biopsy. Indications and methods, *J Dermatol Surg Oncol* **18**: 673–682.

Ronger S, Touzet S, Ligeron C *et al* (2002) Dermoscopical examination of nail pigmentation, *Arch Dermatol* **138**: 1327–33.

Saida T, Ohshima Y (1989) Clinical and histopathologic characteristics of early lesions of subungual malignant melanoma, *Cancer* **63**: 556–560.

Stolz W, Braun-Falco O, Bilek P, Landthaler M, Cognetta AB (1994) Subungual pigmentations. In: *Color Atlas of Dermoscopy*, eds Stolz W, Braun-Falco O, Bilek P, Landthaler M, Cognetta AB (Oxford, Blackwell Scientific) pp. 105–107.

13 Treatment of common nail disorders

Antonella Tosti, Robert Baran, Rodney PR Dawber, Eckart Haneke

Brittle nails • Cosmetic treatment of nail dystrophies • Acute paronychia • Blistering distal dactylitis • Chronic paronychia • Onycholysis • Psoriasis • Lichen planus • Twenty-nail dystrophy • Yellow nail syndrome • Onychogryphosis • Nail biting and onychotillomania • Periungual warts • Further reading

The human nail, chemically similar to horn and hoof, is not essential to the survival of *Homo sapiens*, but it has many important functions that are crucial for the efficient use of the hands and feet. It is also a prime route for the transmission of organisms (both macro- and microscopic), toxins, irritants and allergens. Maintaining nail cleanliness is essential to many aspects of health. Nails of nurses may be the vehicle of transmission of severe and fatal infections, especially in neonatal or intensive care units. Nurses should keep their nails short and avoid wearing artificial nails and nail varnishes.

The nail is also important for beauty; for many people cleanliness alone does not achieve aesthetic satisfaction. A multitude of products, implements and procedures are now on sale to enhance the appearance of nails and finger tips. While the cosmetic industry encourages and caters for the trappings of nail care and adornment, the motivation is probably innate; nail beautification was an established practice in societies long past, and the long finger nail – often accentuated by gold and jewelled fingertip extenders – was indicative of high rank and station in society. Thus

for social, cosmetic and cultural reasons and to aid normal function of digits with abnormal nails it is important to consider cosmetic, podiatric or chiropody treatment for dystrophies in which cure is not possible.

Many nail conditions require camouflage. Several factors should be taken into account:

- the age of the patient
- the sex of the patient
- the type and origin of the dystrophy
- the part of the nail apparatus affected (nail plate or distal phalanx).

BRITTLE NAILS

Nail brittleness causes several clinical symptoms including splitting, softening, lamellar exfoliation and onychorrhexis. Brittle nails are a common complaint. It is often an idiopathic condition, but can also be a symptom of a large number of dermatological nail disorders. Although brittle nails have been linked with many internal diseases, the high frequency of nail fragility in the general population makes it difficult to prove the validity of any such association. Environmental and occupational factors that produce a progressive dehydration of the nail plate play an important part in the development of idiopathic nail brittleness. The lipid content of the nail is influenced by sexual hormones and decreases after menopause. This explains the high prevalence of brittle nails in postmenopausal women.

Management of brittle nails requires preventive and protective measures to avoid nail plate dehydration. Affected individuals should wear cotton gloves under rubber gloves during household tasks, avoid repeated immersion of the hands in soap and water, and keep their nails short. Nail varnishes may be protective, but the use of nail varnish remover should be limited since it exacerbates brittleness. Local therapies are useful in the treatment of nail brittleness. Application of a petroleum jelly preparation on wet nails at bedtime helps to retain the moisture in the nail plate. Frequent topical application of preparations containing hydrophilic substances such as phospholipids, hyaluronic acid, alpha-hydroxy acids and proteoglycans may favour nail plate rehydration.

Nail wrapping limited to the distal portion of the nail may afford protection and camouflage in recalcitrant fragility of the nail keratin. Oral treatment with biotin 2.5 mg per day for several months or even all year round can be useful as it may improve the synthesis of the lipid molecules that produce binding between nail plate corneocytes.

COSMETIC TREATMENT OF NAIL DYSTROPHIES

Cosmetics available for nail treatment include:

- nail varnish and stick-on nail dressing
- preformed artificial nails
- sculptured artificial nails
- nail wrapping

- adaptable nail prostheses
- abrader.

Nail varnish

Nail varnish may hide any type of chromonychia in women (or even girls) if the surface of the nail plate is smooth, or if it can be rendered so by fine sandpaper. The hue resulting from *Pseudomonas* nail infection is often hidden by nail varnish, which may be kept on during the treatment with sodium hypochlorite and is a helpful therapy for this condition. Psoriasis may benefit from the use of nail varnish under some circumstances.

Stick-on nail dressing

Also known as 'press-on nails', this consists of a very thin, coloured synthetic film with an adhesive which fixes it firmly to the nail.

Press-on nails may be used to hide nail discolouration or mild dystrophies. They may cause side effects that vary considerably in intensity from patient to patient: flaking, roughness, ridging, onycholysis, disappearance of the lunula and disorganization of the nail plate which may be delaminated and broken off. Mild paronychial inflammation with loss of the cuticle may be seen.

In some instances 9–12 months will pass before the nails entirely return to normal. The effect on the nail is simply traumatic, not allergic, a combination of the impermeability of the adhering film and the cumulative trauma to the nail plate when the film is repeatedly pulled off.

Preformed artificial nails

Any dystrophy may be hidden by preformed artificial nails, providing that some natural nail plate surface is still present to allow adequate adhesion. It is obvious that a severe dystrophy will prevent this and the usefulness of such a prosthetic nail is then limited. Local complications may appear when preformed artificial nails remain on for 3–4 days.

Distant allergic eczematous contact dermatitis may occur, more often due to the glue than to the prosthetic nail itself.

Sculptured artificial nails

Some natural nail keratin must be present for sculptured artificial nails to be used. The natural nail is first roughened with a burr, then painted with the acrylic resins which harden at room temperature and become moulded on to the nail. The prosthesis can be filed and manicured to shape. As the nail grows out, further applications of the self-curing acrylic resins can be made to maintain a regular contour.

Allergic contact dermatitis may appear, generally after 2–4 months of application, as distant sensitization (face, eyelids) or local reactions (onychial and paronychial tissues). On patch testing, the patient may react strongly to the acrylic liquid monomer.

Nail wrapping

In nail wrapping the free edge of each nail is splinted with layers of a fibrous substance such as cotton wool, paper or plastic film affixed with a variety of glues; after drying, the edge is fashioned to requirements and the nail is coated with enamel. The entire procedure is repeated every 2 weeks. Nail wrapping is useful but can do significant harm if the entire nail is covered because of the occlusive nature of the material used. Allergic reactions to cyanoacrylate nail preparations (painful paronychia, onychodystrophy, discoloration and even exceptional permanent nail loss) are rare, but may persist for more than a year.

Adaptable nail prosthesis

In a wide variety of conditions, ranging from deformed nails to complete loss of the distal phalanx, and in women particularly, a silicone rubber thimble-shaped finger cover may be employed. The fixation is excellent. The device is easy to clean (plain soap), flame-resistant, and the formed nail takes varnish well.

Nail abrasion

Thick nails caused by diseases such as psoriasis, pityriasis rubra pilaris and pachyonychia congenita can be abraded. Hyperkeratosis is prone to be associated with onychomycosis of the toes. Nail abrasion helps to expose the nail bed to antifungal chemicals, especially in elderly people in whom systemic treatment is not advisable. Abrasion is a good way to improve the contour of an abnormal nail, for example in onychogryphosis. In selected cases of ingrowing toe nail, repeated thinning of the nail plate may be a useful conservative method in association with appropriate definitive treatment.

There are many products, implements and devices for maintaining clean, well-groomed nails to satisfy individual needs. These benefits are obtained with small risk. The physician can and should be well versed in nail care and adornment to aid patients in achieving an improved, positive self-image: when specific medical cure is shown to be impossible, the physician will then be in a good position to judge the value of cosmetic, chiropody or podiatry treatments.

ACUTE PARONYCHIA

Acute paronychia is usually caused by *Staphylococcus aureus*, although other bacteria and herpes simplex virus may occasionally be responsible. Minor trauma commonly precedes the infection. Whenever possible cultures should be taken.

Treatment consists of local application of an antiseptic compound such as chlorhexidine or povidone–iodine, and administration of systemic antibiotics. If acute paronychia does not show clear signs of response to penicillinase-resistant antibiotics within 2 days, then surgical treatment should be instituted using proximal block anaesthesia. The base of the nail is removed by cutting across with pointed scissors.

BLISTERING DISTAL DACTYLITIS

Blistering distal dactylitis is a childhood disease usually caused by β hemolytic streptococcus infection, characterized by bullous lesions with purulent content localized at the tip of the digits. Treatment includes surgical drainage of the blisters, topical medication with antiseptics and systemic antibiotics (oral erythromycin or amoxicillin).

CHRONIC PARONYCHIA

Chronic paronychia represents an inflammatory reaction of the proximal nail fold to irritants or allergens. It affects hands that are continually exposed to a wet environment and to multiple microtrauma, favouring cuticle damage. Secondary colonization with *Candida albicans* and/or bacteria occurs in most cases.

Patients with chronic paronychia should avoid a wet environment, chronic microtrauma and contact with irritants or allergens.

Application of high-potency topical steroids (clobetasol propionate 0.05%) once a day at bedtime is an effective first-line therapy. If *Candida* is present a topical imidazole derivative should be applied in the morning. Topical antifungal agents alone and systemic antifungal therapy are not useful. In severe cases, intralesional or even systemic steroids (prednisone 20 mg/day) can be used for a few days to obtain a prompt reduction of inflammation and pain. Acute exacerbations of chronic paronychia do not necessitate antibiotic treatment since they subside spontaneously in a short time. *Pseudomonas* colonization can be treated with sodium hypochlorite solution or 2% acetic acid. Complete recovery of the condition usually requires several weeks and treatment should be continued until the cuticle has regrown. Recurrences are frequent since the barrier function of the proximal nail fold may be impaired for months or even years after an episode of chronic paronychia. In rare cases, foreign bodies such as hair or fibreglass spicules can be responsible for chronic paronychia. These patients should be treated by the excision of a crescent-shaped, full-thickness piece of the proximal nail fold, including its swollen portion. Complete healing by granulation takes about 4 weeks.

ONYCHOLYSIS

Onycholysis (detachment of the nail plate from the nail bed) starts in the central or lateral portion of the nail plate free margin, progresses proximally and can even involve the whole nail. The onycholytic area looks whitish because of the presence of air under the detached nail plate. It may occasionally show a greenish or brown discoloration due to colonization of the onycholytic space by chromogenic bacteria (*Pseudomonas aeruginosa*), moulds or yeasts. Onycholysis may be idiopathic or represent a symptom of numerous diseases (such as psoriasis, onychomycosis or contact dermatitis) or drug reactions.

Depending on the cause of the complaint (e.g. disease or impaired peripheral circulation), appropriate local treatment, systemic treatment or both is prescribed. The detached nail should be clipped away and a mild antibacterial solution (thymol 4% in chloroform) should be applied on the exposed nail bed at night. *Pseudomonas* infection is easily treated by using sodium hypochlorite solution or 2% acetic acid. Accurate drying of the fingers after hand washing is necessary. A hair dryer may be useful for this purpose.

PSORIASIS

Since treatment of nail psoriasis is always disappointing, before treatment is started the individual problems of every patient should be carefully considered, and in particular the degree of discomfort that results from the nail lesions. Reassuring the patient is probably the best approach for isolated nail pitting, oily patches, mild onycholysis and splinter haemorrhages. However, diffuse onycholysis, subungual hyperkeratosis and severe nail plate surface abnormalities may require a positive therapeutic approach.

> **Local therapies of nail psoriasis only rarely induce complete remission of the disease**

When the nail folds are affected, regular application of topical emollients is useful to reduce scaling and prevent self-induced trauma.

Topical steroids, or combinations of topical steroids with salicylic acid and/or retinoic acid, are widely prescribed. Their efficacy is poor, even when applied with occlusive dressing after chemical or mechanical avulsion of the onycholytic nail plate. Long-term application of topical steroids may result in marked atrophy of the soft tissues of the digits or even in focal resorption of the distal phalanges.

A nail lacquer containing 8% clobetasol propionate, formulated to optimize penetration of the drug through the nail plate, has been developed for use in this condition. This topical treatment, which is effective and well tolerated, produces improvement in most cases of nail psoriasis, with effects directly related to the duration of treatment.

Topical calcipotriol is effective when onycholysis and subungual hyperkeratosis are prominent symptoms. Topical tazarotene 0.1% gel has also been used with good results and tolerability in psoriasis. The latter drug is especially effective in reducing onycholysis (in occluded and non-occluded nails) and pitting (in occluded nails).

Topical psoralens followed by exposure to ultraviolet-A (PUVA) are not very effective owing to poor penetration of the UVA through the nail plate, especially when the plate is thickened. However, this treatment may be useful in pustular psoriasis when recurrent pustular lesions have destroyed the nail plate. Intralesional injections of triamcinolone acetonide 10 mg/ml, at a dose of 0.2–0.5 ml per nail, have proved effective in some cases of nail matrix psoriasis. In patients with nail-plate surface abnormalities the steroids should be injected in the nail matrix, whereas in patients with subungual hyperkeratosis the site of injection should be the nail bed. Injections should be repeated monthly for 6 months, then every 6 weeks for the next 6 months and finally every 2 months for 6–12 months. A digital block is sometimes useful to make the treatment less painful, but when several digits are involved, a wrist block may be the appropriate anaesthesia. However, routine use of this treatment is not recommended because of the pain caused by the injections, the local side-effects and recurrence of the nail abnormalities after discontinuation of the therapy. In addition, the efficacy of intralesional steroids in nail matrix psoriasis is limited, with only 50% success in treating nail pits.

Systemic treatment with methotrexate or cyclosporin can clear the nail changes, but this can be recommended only when nail psoriasis is associated with widespread disease or psoriatic arthritis.

Retinoids are of little value in the treatment of nail psoriasis except for hyperkeratotic nails and pustular psoriasis. Oral administration of etretinate or acitretin can even worsen the nail changes owing to the development of nail brittleness, pyogenic granuloma-like lesions and chronic paronychia. Oral photochemotherapy can improve crumbling of the nail plate and psoriatic involvement of the proximal nail fold, but is less effective in nail pitting or subungual hyperkeratosis. Superficial radiotherapy can have a beneficial effect on psoriatic nails but is not recommended because the benefits are short-lived.

Pustular psoriasis of the nail unit usually fails to respond to conventional topical treatments. Local treatment with topical anti-metabolites (mechlorethamine, 1% fluorouracil) is an option, even though results are variable. Systemic steroids, PUVA and cyclosporin can arrest the development of pustular lesions and avoid permanent scarring of the nail apparatus. A study of 46 patients with pustular psoriasis of the nails indicates that systemic retinoids at low dosage (less than 0.5 mg of acitretin per day) are the treatment of choice in patients with multiple nail involvement, whereas topical calcipotriol is the best option for pustular psoriasis limited to one or two nails. Topical calcipotriol is also useful as maintenance therapy in patients who responded to retinoids, in order to prevent recurrence.

LICHEN PLANUS

Specific nail involvement occurs in about 10% of patients with lichen planus and permanent damage of at least one nail occurs in approximately 4% of patients. However, if lichen planus is correctly diagnosed and treated, permanent damage to the nail unit is rare, even where there is diffuse involvement of the nail matrix.

Systemic steroids are effective in treating nail lichen planus: intramuscular triamcinolone acetonide 0.5 mg/kg every month for 2–3 months usually produces recovery of the nail abnormalities. Intralesional injections of triamcinolone acetonide 10 mg/ml represent a possible, but painful, alternative when the disease is limited to a few finger nails. Mild relapses are frequently observed, but recurrences are usually responsive to therapy. Steroid treatment is not useful in pterygium, since the nail matrix cannot be regenerated. Systemic retinoids at dosages suitable for psoriasis are a good alternative.

TWENTY-NAIL DYSTROPHY

Twenty-nail dystrophy, characterized by nail roughness, can be idiopathic or associated with alopecia areata and less often with lichen planus. It is a benign condition that never causes nail scarring. The nail changes usually regress spontaneously in a few years. Reassuring the patient is probably the best approach to this nail disorder. Although topical PUVA can be effective, continuous treatment is required to maintain the results.

YELLOW NAIL SYNDROME

Yellow nail syndrome is an uncommon disorder of unknown aetiology, characterized by the triad of yellow nails, lymphoedema and respiratory tract involvement. Vitamin E at dosages ranging from 600 to 1200 IU daily can induce a complete clearing of the nail changes. Although the mechanism of action of vitamin E in yellow nail syndrome is still unknown, antioxidant properties of alpha-tocopherol may account for its efficacy. A 5% solution of vitamin E in dimethyl sulphoxide produced marked clinical improvement in a double-blind controlled study. The efficacy of topical vitamin E, however, still needs confirmation. Oral itraconazole, 400 mg daily one week a month for several months, or oral flucouazole, may be beneficial in some cases.

ONYCHOGRYPHOSIS

Chemical avulsion of the overgrowing nail plate with urea ointment is useful and provides considerable relief of the patient's discomfort. Different formulations can be used, ranging from a simple 40% urea in 60% white petrolatum preparation, to the South and Farber's ointment, which has the following formulation: urea 40%, white beeswax 5%, anhydrous lanolin 20%, white petrolatum 25%, micronized silica gel 10%. Before the ointment is applied to the nail plate surface, it is mandatory to cover the periungual skin with plastic tape in order to protect the skin from maceration. The urea ointment is then applied to the nail and covered with a plastic wrap; the medication is fixed to the digit with a plastic tape and maintained in place for 7–10 days. Finally, the medication is wiped off and the softened nail plate is removed using nail clippers.

Chemical nail avulsion is only effective when the nail plate is partially or totally detached from the nail bed. It is not useful on normal nails, but can be successful in removing onychomycotic nails as well as thickened psoriatic nails.

NAIL BITING AND ONYCHOTILLOMANIA

Frequent application of distasteful topical preparations on the nail and periungual skin can discourage patients from biting and chewing their finger nails. Possible alternatives include:

- 1% clindamycin
- quaternary ammonium derivatives
- 4% quinine sulphate in petrolatum.

Patients with severe onychophagia or median nail dystrophy can be helped by daily bandaging the injured fingers with permeable adhesive tape. Fluoxetine at high dosages (60 mg/day) can be helpful in interrupting this compulsive disorder in adults.

PERIUNGUAL WARTS

Periungual and subungual warts are usually difficult to treat and frequently recur. The life span of periungual warts may be such that they – and the various treatments – may exceed the patience of both patient and physician! Under such circumstances intelligent placebo therapy may well be appropriate. A great variety of treatments are listed in all pharmacopoeias, reflecting their individually limited success rates. The choice of treatment depends on:

- number of warts
- location (periungual and subungual)
- duration
- age of the patient

- immunological status
- skills of the doctor.

Surgical procedures should be restricted to selected cases.

Topical treatment

Topical agents include: keratolytic agents, virucidal agents and immunomodulators.

Keratolytic agents

Keratolytic agents are the most popular first-line treatment of warts and are particularly suitable for young children, who can apply at home creams, ointments, tapes or quick-drying acrylate lacquers containing salicylic acid in concentrations ranging from 10% to 40%.

Virucidal agents

Both glutaraldehyde and formaldehyde combine with keratin and produce skin desiccation with viral destruction. Effectiveness is comparable to that of keratolytic agents.

Immunotherapy

Topical immunotherapy with strong topical sensitizers – squaric acid dibutylester (SADBE) or diphenylcyclopropenone (DPCP) – is an effective and painless treatment for multiple warts. A preparation of SADBE or DPCP 2% in acetone is used for sensitization. After 21 days weekly applications are carried out with dilutions ranging from 0.001% to 1% according to the patient's response. The objective of treatment is to induce a mild contact dermatitis.

Imiquimod acts as an immunomodulator owing to its capacity to induce cytokine (especially interferon alpha) production. Although imiquimod has only been used for treatment of genital and facial warts, its effectiveness in these regions suggests its possible use for periungual warts.

Systemic treatment

Oral immunomodulators

The efficacy of cimetidine 750–1200 mg per day has never been definitively proved. The drug is expensive and not always well tolerated.

Interferon

The efficacy of interferons is still debated and the necessity of intravenous administration together with cost of treatment do not recommend its routine use. However, complete cure of recalcitrant and extensive periungual and subungual warts has been reported after interferon beta treatment.

Antimitotics

Intralesional injections of bleomycin are effective in the treatment of periungual warts. After local anaesthesia, the bleomycin solution (1 U bleomycin per 1 ml sterile saline) is dropped on the wart surface. The wart is then punctured using a disposable needle approximately 40 times per 5 mm^2 area. The wart slowly undergoes necrosis with formation of an eschar that can be scraped away 3–4 weeks after treatment. Residual warts can be retreated.

Surgical treatment

Cryotherapy

Freezing warts with liquid nitrogen is a rapid method of treatment. It is contraindicated in small children, since it is frequently associated with intense pain secondary to oedema under the nail bed. Application of a surface anaesthetic cream 1–2 hours prior to therapy does not help to reduce pain in the periungual region. Hyperkeratotic warts should be pared off before treatment to permit freezing of the deeper portions of the wart. Freezing takes 10–15 seconds using cryogen spray. A 1 mm halo ring should form in the normal skin surrounding the wart. Cryosurgery should be used with caution for warts on the proximal nail fold, since nail matrix damage is a common complication, with leukonychia, Beau's lines and onychomadesis. Irreversible matrix destruction with nail atrophy has been reported after overzealous cryosurgery.

Surgical excision

Excision of periungual warts is not recommended since it produces scarring and is associated with a high frequency of recurrence.

- Electrosurgery should be avoided, since it produces considerable scarring.
- Infrared coagulation is another destructive method that is not recommended.
- Localized heating using a radiofrequency heat generator has been successfully used to treat hand warts (86% cure). This treatment is not particularly painful, but may cause scarring and does not seem suitable for periungual warts.

Laser techniques

- Carbon dioxide laser: this causes thermic destruction of the wart, producing a loss of skin which heals by secondary intention. When warts extend into the nail folds or the nail bed, laser treatment should be preceded by partial or total nail avulsion. Re-epithelialization takes a long time (approximately 9 weeks) and is associated with risk of infections and pain. Some authors reported complete cures in 71% of patients with periungual warts exclusively treated with one or two sessions of CO_2 laser. Temporary or permanent nail dystrophy were observed in 29% of treated patients. Pain sometimes persists after wound healing. Scarring is not rare, as well as disturbance of function. This technique is suggested only as a secondary approach for recalcitrant warts.
- Pulsed dye laser: this laser acts through a selective microvascular destruction of the dilated capillaries of the warts, since the oxyhaemoglobin contained in the vessels preferentially absorbs yellow light. Healing of the wart is due both to thermic damage and to removal of the blood supply. Stimulation of a cell-mediated immune response may be another contributing factor. A few days after the procedure the wart becomes dry and black, as a result of necrosis. Since no wound is produced, patients may return to work immediately and postoperative pain is minimal. Healing occurs after 2–4 weeks. Periungual warts are less responsive to treatment than palmar or common warts. Although this technique is associated with a very low incidence of scarring, cure is achieved in only a third of cases, and usually after two to four treatments.
- Erbium:YAG laser: the erbium:ytrium–aluminium–garnet (YAG) laser produces a controlled tissue ablation with minimal thermal damage compared with the CO_2 laser. This laser has been used for periungual warts with an excellent safety profile and minimal morbidity and pain.

FURTHER READING

Chronic paronychia

Tosti A, Piraccini BM, Ghetti E *et al* (2002) Topical steroids versus antifungals in the treatment of chronic paronychia: an open, randomized double blind and double dummy study, *J Am Acad Dermatol* **47**: 73–76.

Psoriasis

Baran R, Tosti A (1999) Topical treatment of nail psoriasis with a new corticoid-containing nail lacquer formulation, *J Dermatol Treat* **10**: 201–204.

De Berker D (2000). Management of nail psoriasis, *Clin Exp Dermatol* **25**: 357–362.

Piraccini BM, Tosti A, Iorizzo M *et al* (2001) Pustular psoriasis of the nails: treatment and long-term follow-up of 46 patients, *Br J Dermatol* **144**: 1000–1005.

Scher RK, Stiller M, Zhu YI (2001) Tazarotene 0.1% gel in the treatment of finger nail psoriasis: a double-blind, randomized, vehicle-controlled study, *Cutis* **68**: 355–358.

Lichen planus

Tosti A, Piraccini BM, Cambiaghi S *et al* (2001) Nail lichen planus in children: clinical features, response to treatment and long-term follow-up, *Arch Dermatol* **137**: 1027–1032.

Yellow nail syndrome

Tosti A, Piraccini BM, Iorizzo M (2002) Systemic itraconazole in the yellow nail syndrome. *Br J Dermatol* **146**: 1064–1067.

Baran R (2002). The new oral antifungal drugs in the treatment of the yellow nail syndrome. *Br J Dermatol* **147**: 189–191.

Periungual warts

Tosti A, Piraccini BM (2001) Warts of the nail unit: surgical and non-surgical approach, *Dermatol Surg* **27**: 235–239.

Index

Numbers in italics indicate *tables* or *figures*.

abrasive treatment 227
acquired periungual fibrokeratomas
    95–6
Acremonium spp., routes of nail
    invasion *156*
acrocephalosyndactyly *27*
acrodermatitis enteropathica,
    paronychia in *86*
acrodysostosis *27*
acrokeratosis paraneoplastica
    118–19
acromegaly, clubbed appearance in
    12, *14*
acropustulosis 115–16
acrosclerosis, onychatrophy in *37*
acyclovir 112
Addison's disease *108*
AEC syndrome, micronychia in *31*
alimentary tract disorders and
    clubbing 14–15
alopecia areata
    nail histopathology 193–4
    pitting 55, *56*
    trachyonychia *57*, 59, 60
alopecia unguium 67
Alternaria spp., route of nail invasion
    156
amputation for malignant melanoma
    110
amyloidosis 48, *61*, *123*, 194
anaemia, leukonychia due to 132
anonychia 35, *36–7*
antibiotic treatment for acute
    paronychia 81
antimalarial treatment, nail
    discoloration due to *140*
antimycotic agents 155
aplastic anonychia 35, 69
arched nails *see* pincer nails
artificial nails
    preformed 226–7
    sculptured 227
Aspergillus spp.
    A. candidus WSO *149*
    A. flavus PSO 147
    A. niger onychomycosis *153*

    routes of nail invasion *156*

Bazex syndrome 118–19
Beau's lines
    causes 52–4
    information obtained from 51
    in normal infants 6
benign juvenile digital fibromatosis
    96–7
benign pemphigus (Hailey–Hailey
    disease) *132*, 194
Berk Tabatznik syndrome *27*
bidet nails 34–5
biotin treatment 226
black nails *see* melanonychia (brown
    or black nails)
black superficial onychomycosis
    150
bleomycin *53*, 93, 232
blistering distal dactylitis 114, 228
Bloch–Sulzberger syndrome
    (incontinentia pigmenti) 195–6
blood supply to the nails 4, *5*
blue/grey nails *138*
Bowen's disease 102–3, *108*, 198
brachyonychia (short nails) 22–8
    causes *26*
    clinical picture 22–5, *28*
    hereditary forms *27*
brittle nails 124–5, 225–6
brown nails *see* melanonychia
    (brown or black nails)
Bunell's technique 81
Butcher's nodule 92

calcipotriol 230
calcium in the nail plate 4, 125
callosity (callus) 171
candidal onycholysis 67
candidal onychomycosis 155–8
candidal paronychia 84, 114–15
candidal TDO 150–1
cantharidin 93
carbon dioxide lasers 233
cardiovascular disease and clubbing
    14

chemical nail avulsion 231
chemotherapy, Beau's lines due to
    53
chevron nails 6
children
    benign juvenile digital fibromatosis
        96–7
    blistering distal dactylitis 114,
        228
    chronic paronychia and thumb
        sucking 84, 114–15
    fragility of nail matrix 82
    ingrowing toe nails 175–6
    koilonychia 15, *17*
    nail apparatus 6
    trachyonychia *57*, 59, 60
    Veillonella infections 112–13
chromonychia 127–41
    camouflage of 226
    examination of nails for 127
    factors affecting nail colour 127
    leukonychia *see* leukonychia
        (white nails)
    melanonychia *see* melanonychia
        (brown or black nails)
    other discolorations *138*, 139–40
    see also dermoscopy of nail
        pigmentation
chronic mucocutaneous candidiasis
    156, 157
chronic trauma to the nail
    causative factors
        abnormal foot function 163,
            165
        foot and digit shape 165–7
        footwear *165*, 167–9, 169–70
        old age 169
        reduction of 170
    region affected
        bony phalanx 185
        distal joint 185
        nail apparatus 182–5
        surrounding tissue 171–82
cimetidine 232
clavus 171–3
claw-like nails 29

claw toes *167*
clobetasol propionate nail lacquer
      229
clubbing (Hippocratic fingers) 9–15
   classification
      acquired forms 13–15
      idiopathic forms 12
   diagnostic signs 9, *10*
   general causes *13*
   phalangeal depth ratio
         measurement 9, *10*
   types
      hypertrophic pulmonary
            osteoarthropathy 11
      pachydermoperiostosis 11–12
      simple 10–11
coccal nail-fold angiomatosis 197
congenital onychodysplasia of index
      finger nails (COIF), micronychia
      in 30–1
contact dermatitis, Beau's lines in
      52
copper staining of nails *139*
corns 171–3
cosmetic treatment of nail
      dystrophies 226–7
cryosurgery
   myxoid pseudocysts 102
   warts 93, 233
cuticles *2, 3*
   ragged 88–9
cysts
   keratin 195, 214
   see also myxoid pseudocysts

Darier's disease, nail involvement
      34, 74, 123, 194
dermatofibromas 94
dermatomyositis, ragged cuticles in
      89
dermoscopy of nail pigmentation
      217–23
   diagnostic applications
      drug-induced pigmentation 221
      ethnic nail pigmentation 221–2
      lentigines 220–1
      melanocytic naevi *219,* 220
      melanomas *218,* 220
      subungual haemorrhages 222
   equipment 217
   semiological patterns 217–20
   usefulness of 217
diphencyprone 93
diphenylcyclopropenone (DPCP)
      232

distal lateral subungual
      onychomycosis (DLSO) 143–6,
      151, 192
distal nail embedding 180–2
dolichonychia (long nails) 22, *23*
DOOR syndrome, anonychia in 35,
      36
dorsolateral fissures of the finger tip
      90
DPCP (diphenylcyclopropenone)
      232
dyskeratosis congenita 125
dyskeratosis follicularis *see* Darier's
      disease, nail involvement

eczema
   nail histopathology 194
   nail pitting 56
eggshell nails 123
elastodysplasia 97
elkonyxis 61
endocrine disorders and clubbing
      15
endonyx onychomycosis 150, *151,*
      192
epidermoid carcinomas 102–4, 198
epidermoid cysts, MRI of 214
epidermolysis bullosa, onychatrophy
      in *38, 39*
erbium:YAG lasers 233
erosions (pits) 54–6, 192–3
etretinate therapy and nail disorders
   chronic paronychia *86*
   nail fragility 122
   onychatrophy *37*
exostoses, subungual 99–100, 197

familial mandibuloacral dysplasia *27*
fibromas
   acquired periungual fibrokeratomas
      95–6, 196
   benign juvenile digital
         fibromatoses 96–7
   dermatofibromas 94
   keloids 94
   Koenen's tumours 94–5, 196
   matrix 196
   subungual filamentous tumours
      96, 196
finger nails
   factors controlling shape 1
   growth rates 6
finger/thumb sucking 84, 114–15
fissures, finger tip 90
fluconazole 155

foot digit deformities
   hallux rigidus 166
   hallux valgus 165–6
   lesser digits 166–7
foot function
   abnormal 163, 165
   corrective orthoses 170
   normal gait cycle 163, *164*
footwear and nail problems
   occupational 169–70
   shoe design
      fastenings 168
      heel height 167–8
      seams 169
      toe box dimensions *165,*
         168–9
fragile nails 121–5
Fraser's nail brace technique 179
Fusarium spp.
   F. oxysporum paronoychia 84
   onychomycoses *148, 149*
   routes of nail invasion *156*

garlic clove' fibromas 95, *96*
glomus bodies 4
glomus tumours
   clinical picture *48,* 97–8, *188*
   histopathology 98, 197
   MRI *203,* 206–11
   treatment 98–9
   ultrasonography 202, *203*
glycoprotein 63–4
green nails *138,* 139, *140*
grey/blue nails *138*
griseofulvin 155

haematological causes of clubbing
      15
haematomas *see* subungual
      haematomas
Hailey–Hailey disease *132,* 194
half-and-half nails 131–2
half-moons (lunulae) 1, *2*
Hallopeau's disease 115–16
hallux rigidus 166
hallux valgus 165–6
hammer toes *167*
hand, foot and mouth disease 195
hangnails 88, *89,* 182
hapalonychia 121, 123
hard nails 121
Heller's median canaliform dystrophy
      48, 49
herpes simplex infections
   clinical picture 111–12, *187*

differential diagnosis 112
histopathology 194–5
and thumb/finger sucking 115
treatment 112
herpes zoster infections 112, *188*, 195
herringbone nails 51, *52*
hidrotic ectodermal dysplasia, micronychia in *31*
Hippocratic fingers *see* clubbing (Hippocratic fingers)
histopathology of nail disorders 191
see also specific disorders
Hjorth–Sabouraud syndrome 117–18, 194
hook-like nails 29–30, 163
Hutchinson's sign 107, 220
micro-Hutchinson's sign *218*, 220
see also pseudo-Hutchinson's sign
hyperkeratosis
callus 171
complications of 173
corns 171–3
treatment 173–4
hypertrophic lateral nail fold 176, *177*
hypertrophic pulmonary osteoarthropathy 11
hypertrophy of the nail plate 70
hypoalbuminaemia, Muehrcke's lines 130–1

idiopathic hypertrophic osteoarthropathy (pachydermoperiostosis) 11–12
imaging of the nail unit
MRI *see* magnetic resonance imaging (MRI) of the nail unit
radiography 201–2
ultrasonography 202–4
imiquimod 232
immunotherapy for warts 232
impetigo 113
incontinentia pigmenti 195–6
ingrowing toe nails 175–6
interferon treatment for warts 232
involuted nails *see* pincer nails
iron deficiency 125
Iso–Kikuchi syndrome (COIF), micronychia in 30–1
isotretinoin therapy, chronic paronychia due to *86*
itraconazole 155, 158

jogger's toe 171

Keipert syndrome *27*
keloids 94
keratin cysts 195, 214
keratinocytes, nail matrix 3
keratin structure changes in nail disorders 124–5
keratoacanthomas 97, 195, 214
keratolytic agents 232
keratosis cristarum 73
keratosis follicularis *see* Darier's disease, nail involvement
ketoconazole 155, 158
Koenen's ungual fibromas 94–5, 196
koilonychia (spoon-shaped nails) 15–18

lamellar splitting (onychoschizia) 60–2, *122*
Larsen's syndrome *27*
laser therapy for warts 233
Laugier–Hunziker–Baran syndrome *105*, *108*, 221
lentigines 220–1
leprosy, leukonychia in 132
leukonychia (white nails) 128–34
apparent leukonychia
Muehrcke's lines 130–1
Neapolitan nails 132
Terry's nails 130
uraemic half-and-half nails 131–2
causes summarized *133*
dermatoses causing 132–3
pseudoleukonychia 134
true leukonychia
isolated longitudinal 130
leukonychia variegata 130
punctate 130
subtotal 129
total 128
transverse 129–30, 184, *185*
types summarized 128
lichen planus of the nails
histopathology 193
longitudinal lines *46*, 47
nail fragility *122*
onychatrophy *40*
onychorrhexis *61*
onychoschizia 61
subungual hyperkeratosis *74*
trachyonychia 58, *59*
treatment 230

lichen striatus of the nails 193
liquid nitrogen treatment *see* cryosurgery
LM *see* longitudinal melanonychia (LM)
longitudinal lines
causes *51*
grooves 45–50
ridges 51
longitudinal melanonychia (LM) 104
causes *105*, *135*
malignant melanomas *see* malignant melanomas of the nail region
melanocyte activation 104–5
melanocyte hyperplasia 105–6
nail matrix naevi 106
see also melanonychia (brown or black nails)
long nails (dolichonychia) 22, *23*
Lovibond's profile sign 11
lung cancer, clubbing in 10
lunulae (half-moons) 1, *2*
lupus erythematosus *87*, 193
Lyell's syndrome, nail shedding in 67, *68*

macronychia 30, 32
magnetic resonance imaging (MRI) of the nail unit 204–15
coils 204
positioning of the patient 204–5
routine examination 205
tumour diagnosis
epidermoid cysts 214
glomus tumours *203*, 206–11
keratoacanthomas 214
myxoid pseudocysts 211–14
onychomatricomas *205*, 215
vascular tumours 211
malignant melanomas of the nail region 106–10
amelanotic 107, *109*
dermoscopy of *218*, 220
differential diagnosis *91*, 107–9, 138
features indicative of 138
histopathology 110, 198
LM as initial sign 106
pigmented, characteristics of 107
prognosis 110
tissue diagnosis guidelines 109–10
treatment 110
mallet toes *167*

Marfan's syndrome, dolichonychia in
    23
matrix fibromas   196
median nail dystrophy   *48*, 49
melanocytes, nail matrix   3
    activation   104–5
    hyperplasia   105–6
melanocytic naevi   106, 197–8
    dermoscopy of   *219*, 220
melanomas, malignant *see* malignant
    melanomas of the nail region
melanonychia (brown or black nails)
    134–9
    causes   *135*, 183
    dangers of misdiagnosis   138,
        139
    features indicative of melanoma
        138, 217
    frictional   183, *184*
    longitudinal *see* longitudinal
        melanonychia (LM)
    potassium permanganate staining
        138, 139
    silver nitrate staining   *137*, 139
melanosomes   105
micro-Hutchinson's sign   *218*, 220
micronychia   30–2
MRI *see* magnetic resonance
    imaging (MRI) of the nail unit
mucoid cysts *see* myxoid
    pseudocysts
Muehrcke's lines   130–1
multicentric reticulohistiocytosis
    197
myxoid pseudocysts
    clinical picture   100–1
    histopathology   101, 196–7
    MRI   *186*, 211–14
    treatment   101–2

naevi *see* melanocytic naevi
nail
    abrasion   227
    apparatus
        blood supply   4, *5*
        in childhood   6
        function   1
        microscopic anatomy   3–4
        nerve supply   4, *5*
        in old age   6–7
        structure   1–3
    artefacts   182
    beds   3–4
    biting   231
    brace techniques   179–80

colour changes *see* chromonychia
consistency *see* nail consistency
dynamics
    cell kinetics   4–5
    linear nail growth   6
folds   1–2, 3
matrices   2, 3, 4–5
pits   54–6, 192–3
plates
    in childhood   6
    function   1
    microscopic anatomy   4
    in old age   7
    production   5
    reasons for flat growth   5
    zones   3
prostheses   227
pustulation
    conditions causing   *111*
    see also specific conditions
shedding   67–70, 160, 183
varnish
    nail fragility due to   *122*
    to camouflage chromonochias
        226
    for treatment of nail psoriasis
        229
water content of   124
wrapping   50, 227
nail consistency   121–5
    fragile/brittle/soft nails
        associated conditions   121, 123
        causes   124–5
        morphological types   124
        treatment (brittle nails)   225–6
    hard nails   121
nail–patella syndrome   29, 35, *37*,
    51, *52*
nanocephalic dwarfism   *27*
Neapolitan nails   132
Neisseria gonorrhoeae pustules
    112
nerves to the nails   4, *5*

oil patches   64
old age, nails in   6–7, *45*, *46*
omega nails *see* pincer nails
onychatrophy   35, *37–42*
onychia punctata (pits)   54–6, 192–3
Onychocola canadensis, route of nail
    invasion   *156*
onychocryptosis
    distal nail embedding   180–2
    hypertrophy of the lateral lip
        176, *177*

juvenile ingrowing toe nail   175–6
pincer nails *see* pincer nails
types   174–5
onychodermal bands   3
onychogryphosis   *71*
    causes   70, *72*
    treatment   231
onycholemmin horns   195
onycholysis
    causes   65–7, 174
    clinical picture   63–4, 228
    patterns of separation   63
    in psoriasis   63–4
    of the toe nails   65, 67
    treatment   229
    types   64–5
onychomadesis   51, *53*, 67–70, 174
onychomatricomas
    clinical signs   93–4
    histopathology   94, 196, 215
    MRI   *205*, *206*, 215
onychomycosis   143–58
    candidal   155–8
    causes   *143*
    diagnosis
        collection of specimens   151–2
        culture   152, 154
        histopathology   152, 191–2
    differential diagnosis   154–5
    routes of nail invasion   143, *156*
    treatment   155
    types
        distal lateral subungual   143–6
        endonyx   150, *151*
        proximal subungual   146, *147–8*
        superficial   146, *148–9*, 150
        total dystrophic   150–1
onychophosis   173
onychoptosis defluvium   67
onychorrhexis   47–8, *61*
onychoschizia (lamellar splitting)
    60–2, *122*
onychotillomania   *41–2*, 49, 183,
    231
orthoses   170
osteochondroma   99–100
otopalatodigital syndrome   *27*

pachydermoperiostosis   11–12
pachyonychia congenita   *73*
painful nails   185–9
parakeratosis pustulosa   117–18, 194
paronychia   81–8
    acute
        causes   81, *85*, 115, 160

differential diagnosis 83
  treatment 81–2, 160, *187*, 228
chronic *86–8*
  acute exacerbations 83–4
  in athletes 182
  causes 83, 84, *85*
  clinical picture 83, 84, 114–15
  differential diagnosis 84
  treatment 84–5, 228
parrot-beak nails 28
pemphigoid *38*, 194
pemphigus, benign familial
  (Hailey–Hailey disease) *132*, 194
pemphigus vulgaris 194
periungual warts *see* warts,
  periungual and subungual
pertinax bodies 4, 7
Peutz–Jeghers syndrome *108*
phalangeal depth ratio measurement
  9, *10*
photo-onycholysis 64, *65*
pincer nails
  causes 20–2
  clinical picture 19–20
  pain 20, 176, 178
  treatment
    conservative management
      178–9
    Haneke's technique 180
    nail brace techniques 179–80
  types 178
pitting 54–6, 192–3
pityriasis rubra pilaris 193
pleonosteosis *27*
plicatured nails 22
Plummer–Vinson syndrome 15
polydactyly 33
potassium permanganate staining of
  nails *138*, 139
press-on nails 226
proximal subungual onychomycosis
  (PSO) 146, *147–8*, 151, 192
pseudoclubbing *13, 14, 27*
pseudo-Hutchinson's sign 107, *108*
pseudohypoparathyroidism *27*
pseudoleukonychia 134
Pseudomonas aeruginosa infections
  139, *140*, 228
pseudo yellow nail syndrome,
  transverse overcurvature in *21*
PSO *see* proximal subungual
  onychomycosis (PSO)
psoriasis of the nails
  Beau's lines *53*, 54
  histopathology 192–3

onychatrophy *39*
onycholysis 63, *64*
onychomadesis *69*
pitting 55, *56*, 192–3
pustular *69*, 115–16, 230
subungual hyperkeratosis *71*
treatment
  intralesional steroid injections
    229–30
  systemic 230
  topical 229
psoriatic arthropathy, brachyonychia
  in *28*
pterygium
  causes *79*, 162
  dorsal 77–9
  treatment 230
  ventral 79
pulsed dye lasers 233
puretic syndrome *27*
purple nails *138*
pustular psoriasis *69*, 115–16, 230
pustules
  conditions with 111
  see also specific conditions
pyogenic granulomas 161

racquet nails *24*, 25, *27*
radiography of the nail unit 201–2
ragged cuticles 88–9
recurring digital fibrous tumours
  96–7
red nails *138*, 140
Reiter's syndrome 116–17, 193
retinoid therapy (oral)
  chronic paronychia due to *86*
  etretinate *see* etretinate therapy
    and nail disorders
  nail psoriasis 115, 230
  onychoschizia due to 61, *62*
  Reiter's syndrome 117
retracted toes *167*
retronychia 67, 69
rheumatoid arthritis, longitudinal nail
  lines *46*
rippled nails 54–5
Rosenau's depressions (pits) 54–6,
  192–3
rough nails *see* trachyonychia (rough
  nails; twenty-nail dystrophy)
round fingerpad sign 28, *29*
Rubinstein–Taybi syndrome *23, 27*

SADBE (squaric acid dibutylester)
  232

sarcoidosis
  onychatrophy due to *38*
  paronychia due to *88*
'sausage link' appearance *46*
scleroderma
  fingerpad sign *29*
  ragged cuticles *89*
Scopulariopsis brevicaulis 153
  routes of nail invasion *156*
scurvy, splinter haemorrhages due to
  75
self-induced trauma *50*, 54, 65,
  182–3
  see also onychotillomania
shedding of nails 67–70, 160, 183
shiny nails 34–5
shoes *see* footwear and nail
  problems
short nails *see* brachyonychia (short
  nails)
silver nitrate staining of nails *137*,
  139
simple clubbing 10–11
Sneddon–Wilkinson disease 116
soft nails 121, 123
solehorns 2
South and Farber's ointment 231
Spiegler tumours 25, *27*
splinter haemorrhages 75–6, *78*,
  160
spoon-shaped nails (koilonychia)
  15–18
sportsman's toe 171
squamous cell carcinoma 103–4,
  198
squaric acid dibutylester (SADBE)
  232
staphylococcal infections, impetigo
  113
Steel's 'garlic clove' fibromas 95,
  96
steroids, topical 229
Stevens–Johnson syndrome,
  onychatrophy after *38*
stick-on nail dressings 226
streptococcal infections
  blistering distal dactylitis 114,
    228
  impetigo 113
subcutaneous ingrowing nails
  175–6
subungual corns 171–3
subungual exostoses 99–100, 197
subungual filamentous tumours 96,
  196

subungual haematomas
  associated conditions *78*
  clinical picture 76–7, *136,*
    159–60
  differentiation from melanomas
    77, 107, 109
  drainage techniques 77
  non-migrating 77
  total 77, 160
subungual haemorrhages
  dermoscopy of 222
  jogger's toe 171
  tennis toe 171
subungual hyperkeratosis 70–4
subungual warts *see* warts,
    periungual and subungual
superficial onychomycosis 146,
    148–9, 150, 192
surgical treatments
  distal nail embedding 180–2
  glomus tumours 98–9
  Haneke's technique for pincer
    nails 180
  ingrowing toe nails 175–6
  paronychia 81–2, 85
  warts 93, 233
  Winograd procedure 176, *177*
  see also cryosurgery
synovialomas 197

TDO (total dystrophic
    onychomycosis) 150–1, 192
tennis toe 171
terbinafine 155
Terry's nails 130
thick nails, causes of *74*
thoracic disorders and clubbing 13
thumb/finger sucking 84, 114–15
thumb polydactyly 33
tile-shaped nails 22
tinea cruris *145,* 146
toe nails
  factors controlling shape 1
  growth rates 6
  ingrowing 175–6

total dystrophic onychomycosis
    (TDO) 150–1, 192
Touraine–Solente–Golé syndrome
    12
trachyonychia (rough nails; twenty-
    nail dystrophy) 56–60
  in alopecia areata *57,* 59, 60
  associations 59, *60*
  causes summarized *60*
  idiopathic *57,* 59
  opaque *58,* 59–60
  shiny *57,* 59, 60
  treatment 230
  transverse lines *see* Beau's lines
  transverse overcurvature 18–22
    common causes *18*
    pincer nails *see* pincer nails
    plicatured nails 22
    tile-shaped nails 22
traumatic disorders of the nail
    159–89
  major
    conditions produced by trauma
      159–61
    delayed effects 161–3
    pain resulting from *186*
    repeated microtrauma *see* chronic
      trauma to the nail
treatment of nail disorders
  cosmetic 226–7
  see also specific disorders
triamcinolone acetonide injections
    229, 230
Trichophyton rubrum
  in culture *154*
  DLSO *144, 145*
  melanonychia *145*
  subungual hyperkeratosis *72*
Trichophyton soudanense 150,
    151, 154
trumpet nails *see* pincer nails
tuberculosis cutis verrucosa
    (butcher's nodule) 92
tumours and swellings of the nail
    unit *90, 91, 92, 186*

see also specific lesions
turf toe 182
twenty-nail dystrophy *see*
    trachyonychia (rough nails;
    twenty-nail dystrophy)

ultrasonography of the nail unit
    202–4
ultraviolet radiation (UV) 7
uraemic half-and-half nails of Lindsay
    131–2
urea ointment 231
usure des ongles 34–5

Veillonella infection in the newborn
    112–13
virucidal agents 232
vitamin C deficiency, splinter
    haemorrhages due to *75*
vitamin E treatment 231

walking, normal gait cycle 163,
    164
warts, periungual and subungual
  clinical picture 90, *91,* 92
  treatment 93, 231–3
  washboard' nail plates 50
water content of nails 124
white nails *see* leukonychia (white
    nails)
white superficial onychomycosis
    (WSO) 146, *148–9,* 150, 152,
    192
Winograd procedure 176, *177*
worn-down nails 34–5

yellow nails *138, 139*
yellow nail syndrome *139*
  hard nails 121
  pseudoclubbing *14*
  transverse overcurvature *20, 21*
  treatment 231

zinc deficiency, paronychia due to
    88